CW00591709

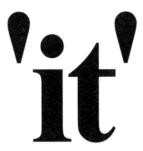

'it'

A wife's journey through....

Jill Lamède

ROUGHTOR
PRESS

Copyright © 1996 Jill Lamède

ISBN 0 9530905 0 7

Published by RoughTor Press, Penhale, Trewarmett,
Tintagel, Cornwall PL34 0ET

First Edition 1997
Cover design by Richard K Beales
Cover photograph by Henry Israel

Printed by Penwell Limited,
Station Road, Kelly Bray, Callington, Cornwall

A.I.D.S. . . . If only he could make himself write down those four letters then, he was sure, he could go on writing, could express some of the pain, anger and terror that had taken over his life.

But RT never managed to write that word. He was a journalist and this ultimate writer's block hurt him deeply. He told me that it would be my task to try to make sense of the ending of his life and to tell the world as best I could.

And so I now set out to tell my husband's story. There is little comfort in it but I hope it may, in some way, help others who are suffering similar torments to know that they are not alone. Certainly there is much for health workers and care providers to learn - so many mistakes made amongst all the good intentions . . .

CHAPTER 1

1994

Let's get one thing clear from the start. RT was not 'at risk'. He was not homosexual or bisexual. He never used drugs or prostitutes. He embraced the concept of 'Safe Sex' as soon as it was invented - but that was too late.

Following a terrible car crash in 1969, where he was at first left lying in the gutter, presumed dead, he did have a massive blood transfusion. Could some of that blood have been infected? The doctors say no, but research is now showing that there may be twenty years or more between the date of infection and the onset of AIDS.

If it was not the blood, then, an even more frightening thought, it must have been just the normal, heterosexual behaviour of a good looking and charming bachelor in the sexually liberated '70s, before we had even heard of HIV.

With hindsight RT was able to recall that the first symptoms started in 1980. There was nothing very dramatic, just some night sweats, increasing tiredness, a bit of tightness in the chest. He put it down to overindulgence in alcohol and tobacco, overwork, lack of exercise and encroaching middle-age. He didn't choose to change his lifestyle and the symptoms recurred from time to time over the next twelve years.

Then he was hit by the recession. He lost his business, his home and his self-respect. His health soon deteriorated. At first it was just a general malaise and increasing exhaustion. The GP sent him to a consultant who had little sympathy. A middle-aged journalist who drinks and smokes? - It must be self-induced liver disease and serve him right. But the liver scan seemed clear.

In December 1993 RT went down with 'flu. The fever and sweating were frightening but he refused to see a doctor and slowly recovered, only to develop a urine infection which did demand medical attention and a course of antibiotics.

By now it was 1994 - a year I shall never forget. A second consultant, not believing the scan, ordered a liver biopsy. RT was frightened. He, too, was sure he had damaged his liver but the biopsy and scan together proved that his liver was large and healthy. So what was making him feel so ill all the time? Consultant no.2 ordered a mass of blood tests. They were all clear, so he ordered some more. All RT was told was, "Well, at least your immune system is all right." That was some comfort but, with no diagnosis, there was no treatment and we were sent away believing it was all in his mind.

But still, arthritic pains were keeping him awake at night and the occasional night-sweats would soak the bed. He had severe indigestion most of the time. There was the fungal infection, called thrush or candida, in his mouth and weeping cracks at the corners of his lips. His sinuses were blocked and catarrh was making him cough. He was exhausted and irritable. His hands and feet were cold. And his anus was itching. Not surprisingly he seemed to be depressed.

The symptoms slowly got worse. By May there was an open wound around his anus. He had seen four doctors but still there was no diagnosis or treatment. They didn't seem to believe that RT was ill, but that might have been his own fault. He would insist on being brave in public. He would always stride into the consulting room, crack jokes and refuse to complain about his many symptoms. He didn't want to make a fuss.

In July the consultant, after noticing a marked weight loss and an increase in the size of the anal wound, confidently diagnosed Crohn's Disease, an incurable condition affecting the digestive system, especially the bowels. RT was horrified. It is such an undignified disease. But I was pleased - at least he could now get some treatment and might start to feel better.

August - another consultant and a second diagnosis of Crohn's. Then a biopsy and no sign of Crohn's Disease. It had been another wrong diagnosis.

By now RT's bottom was in an appalling state. We could hear the doctor gasp in surprise. The wound had spread over most of RT's buttocks and he could not sit down. Opening his bowels was agony. He had been prescribed suppositories and I would find him lying on the bathroom floor in tears, unable to move, after trying to insert them through the raw and weeping flesh. The wound obviously extended inside the rectum.

Driving to the hospital for his next appointment was a nightmare. It was 50 miles of narrow country lanes and for RT there was no position that did not hurt. We arrived to find there would be a delay of two hours and an officious nurse kept insisting that RT should sit down! Nearly in tears, I explained the problem and we were seen by the Registrar. He took one look at the wound and rushed out of the room to fetch the consultant who calmly suggested treating it as a burn.

RT was supposed to lie on his stomach for one month to allow fresh air to reach his bottom - and that was all, no diagnosis just some antibiotics, antidepressants and vitamin pills.

And so we waited for things to improve. They didn't. RT's mouth was full of ulcers. He had frequent nosebleeds and a sore was developing under a nostril. His legs were covered in insect bites that itched all the time and wouldn't heal. The glands in his groin felt small and hard, but didn't hurt. He was becoming clumsy, losing his balance and generally felt very ill indeed. In September the consultant admitted defeat and transferred RT to a skin specialist, promising that he would have an appointment within a week.

But somehow the hospital managed to lose RT's papers and no appointment was made. After many angry and sometimes tearful phone calls we finally got to see the skin specialist in mid-October. He was clearly impressed by size of RT's wounds and asked to take photographs for publication.

He could offer no diagnosis but wanted to do another lot of blood

tests. He asked casually if we would mind if he included an HIV test
amongst them. Why should we mind? We had already been told RT's
immune system was fine and we knew he was not at risk.

Another two weeks of waiting. Another two weeks of no effective
treatment. Another two weeks of steadily worsening symptoms and
increasing despair. RT's mouth was so sore that he had not been eating
properly for months. Now he was managing about a pint of milk a day
and that was all. His weight was dropping fast.

We returned to the hospital. This time the skin specialist seemed
cold and unfriendly. He said that he had some of the blood test results
and that he wanted to repeat one of them and take a new one. That
appeared to be the end of the conversation as far as he was concerned.
RT and I looked at each other. We were determined not to be sent home
yet again to just wait while the symptoms got worse and RT got thinner.
And so RT asked about the HIV test - it was the only one that had a
name we knew.

The consultant replied, "That's the one. I want to do it again."

RT pressed him, "Why? What does it mean? Have I got it?"

"Yes, it's showing positive. I want to do it again and a blood cell
count. Nurse, take them for blood tests - you had better put a High Risk
sticker on the envelope. I'll give you a ring in a few days. Goodbye."

In a state of shock we followed the nurse, had the tests and tried to
drive home.

How can I begin to explain the emotions of that year? RT and I had
been together since the end of 1988. Right from the start I knew that
something was wrong. Like RT I assumed it was just a surfeit of
alcohol combined with overwork.

At that time he was struggling to start his own monthly publication
and was single-handedly writing all the articles, taking the photos,
planning the layouts and selling the adverts. I tried to control the office

and do the accounts, typing and sub-editing in my spare time. Together we worked far too hard - often right through the night to meet the printer's deadline. We were exhausted but proud of our beautiful newspapers.

Then came the recession and the end of our dreams. The business folded. RT's cottage was sold to pay off some of the debts and he moved in with me on a permanent basis. For the first time in his career he had to suffer the indignity of attending the Job Centre and asking for Income Support. He found it hard to bear and I hated to see his pride take such a beating.

Every day he seemed a little more tired, more depressed and he started to complain of feeling unwell. As the symptoms worsened and the doctors failed to provide any diagnosis, despair set in. Most of the time he was in great pain, both physical and emotional. I had to watch the man I loved slowly falling to pieces.

At night I would massage his aching joints and gently knead the muscles of his buttocks to ease the pain of that ugly wound. It looked like a massive ulcer, about 10 inches in diameter, and had spread a little further every night.

By day he would slowly work in the garden, building walls, creating flower beds, in solitary silence, until it was time to go to the pub to try to numb his brain with alcohol.

As soon as I had realised that his pride was preventing him from letting the doctors know just how ill he felt I started to go into the consulting rooms with him. I gave each doctor a written list of all the current symptoms and how they had progressed since the last visit. But still we got no diagnosis.

Of course we had considered HIV. Sometimes RT would say bleakly, "What if I've got 'it'?" I replied that it was a problem we would deal with if and when it happened, but research in the library reassured me that at that time no more than a handful of cases of heterosexual transmission had been found and those were usually women infected by bisexual men. We even discussed it with our GP and he assured us that RT was definitely not at risk - and besides, the consultant had said that

RT's immune system was fine. I wonder what he meant?

And then, at last, the diagnosis. After a whole year of increasing pain and misery, a brutal death sentence with no warning, no counselling, no help, no comfort.

I remember looking at RT. We could not speak. I could hardly see - suddenly I had tunnel vision and could see only a small area directly ahead. Everything else was blood red.

Outside the hospital we stood in the rain and RT asked, "Does this make me a different person?" Misunderstanding him, I replied, "Yes."

I meant that this shock and this illness would, inevitably, change him. But he had been asking if I now would reject him, would cease to love him because he had the 'Gay Plague'.

In silence I drove towards home, 50 miles away. I was aware that I was in shock and not fit to drive but we had to get home somehow. We stopped at a quiet pub and sat holding hands, still in silence. Then RT said, "Would there be any advantage for you if we were married?" - A strange proposal! I promised to research the matter and we sat in silence again. Then he formally apologised to me for being such a burden and thanked me for all my support and help.

My heart was breaking and I can recall nothing more of that nightmare journey home.

RT forbade me to tell anyone of the diagnosis. It must be completely secret - he simply could not cope if anyone found out. And so I had to pretend. I had to tell my mother, who lived next door, that the test results were looking good and that he would soon be getting better. I found the strain of lying intolerable but RT was in such a state of shock that he could not see my distress or understand my need for support.

He had me to talk to, and he talked non-stop. But he was unable to listen and so I had no outlet for my pain. I could feel the pressure building and knew I might explode in rage or collapse completely.

My researches showed that many matters, both bureaucratic and financial, would be easier to handle if I were his next-of-kin. So we decided to marry, very quietly, just before Christmas.

At last I persuaded RT that, for my sake, my mother must be told the truth and together we gave her the bad and the good news - the terminal disease and the wedding in three days time. She responded, as I knew she would, with a calm control, loving support and pleasure that we should be married at last. But there was also anger that she had been excluded from sharing our painful knowledge for so long. She found it hard to forgive RT for adding total secrecy to my burdens.

But it wasn't total. I had recognised my need to share and had selected a few trustworthy friends, who did not live locally, in whom I could confide by telephone when RT was asleep. They provided the essential support that got me through those early days and, as far as I know, none of them betrayed my confidence.

The skin specialist did telephone after five days. The second HIV test had proved positive, the cell count was very low and an appointment had been arranged at the G.U. clinic in seven days' time at 7.30pm.

This message really made little sense to me so I simply agreed and went to look up the meaning of G.U. It stood for Genito-Urinary - the sexually transmitted diseases clinic, the place where embarrassed patients try to slip in unnoticed and unrecognised. It would be another blow to RT's damaged pride.

It had been difficult enough for him to admit to having a sore on his anus. It had been weeks before he allowed me to look at it and he had hated having to expose his posterior to the examination and muffled exclamations of so many doctors.

I rang the G.U. clinic to explain that RT was much too ill to cope with an evening appointment 50 miles away from home and that we were so distraught that we could not handle another seven days of no information or treatment. The receptionist was most understanding and arranged a special late morning appointment for the next day. It was the first sign of positive help we had received.

RT dressed formally for the occasion, as always, tweed suit, M.C.C. tie, gold cufflinks, beautifully polished brogues, but his face was grey and he was so weak that he could scarcely walk. Our progress from the car park, uphill to the clinic, was painfully slow. And then into a small waiting room full of embarrassed men. This was the male clinic day and they had not expected to see a woman walk in.

To be fair, as soon as the receptionist realised who we were she ushered us into a staff room for some privacy. The doctor had been delayed but a counsellor brought us coffee and started to talk to us to try to ease some of the tension we obviously displayed.

The counsellor, like so many people we were to meet from then on, seemed a little hesitant at first. She obviously had not expected to find us such a respectable middle-aged couple.

Eventually the doctor arrived and welcomed us warmly. Once again RT had to drop his trousers and we could hear the doctor gasp, "Oh my God!" as he saw the appalling state of RT's behind.

He talked at length about the virus but he spoke very quietly and it was difficult to follow for both RT and I had hearing problems. While RT was out of the room the doctor put a hand on my arm and said, "You do realise that he could die at any time?"

He explained to us about the cell count - that a normal, healthy adult male would usually have about 1200 CD4 cells and that RT only had 20.

He told us that RT already had advanced AIDS and that there was little he could do but try to ease the worst of the symptoms. He prescribed massive doses of a large number of pills and food supplements, telling RT to drink and smoke as much as he liked.

We were introduced to the various nurses and community workers who would be helping us, shown a private backdoor to the clinic for our future use and given an appointment for two weeks hence.

Without hope we returned home - back to the lies and lonely despair. It was AIDS Awareness Week and we felt obliged to watch every television programme on the subject. They left RT convinced that he would soon be a blind, incontinent and senile skeleton trapped in a wheelchair.

We had been given no literature to read, no contact numbers to ring. We were on our own again trying to cope with the unthinkable.

I wondered whether RT would still be alive for our wedding and went to see the Registrar to find out about a Special Licence in case we should need it. I searched the phone book for suitable sources of information and started asking for help. I needed to be doing something and all this essential research and endless form-filling helped to keep me sane.

I went to the D.S.S. office to try to determine what Benefits we could claim and encountered unfeeling, inefficient bureaucracy at its worst. I asked for a meeting in private, but to the D.S.S. that means simply having a plank of wood screening your face from the client in the next cubicle.

There was a thick sheet of glass between me and the civil servant so that, still in shock and near to tears, I had to speak loudly and strain to hear any replies. I asked to speak to someone who knew about both Income Support and Disability Benefits but was told there was no such person - I could see two different people separately and only deal with one subject at a time. Inevitably the information and forms I received were wrong.

As soon as I got home I rang the D.S.S. freephone advice number and was immediately given accurate information and sympathetic advice.

The medication started to work almost at once. Five days later, when the special Community Nurse came to advise us on how to clean and protect RT's buttocks, they had already begun to heal, as had the sore under his nostrils. His mouth was improving and his strength increasing steadily. When we returned to the clinic he was walking tall and, once again, putting on a brave act, pretending that he felt quite well. Everyone was amazed at the transformation.

If only he had been given that medication months earlier, when the symptoms first appeared. He would have been spared so much pain and despair. But that is the price he had to pay for being heterosexual. There is a cruel, inverted prejudice that means that if he had been younger, less respectable and educated, obviously gay or even just single, he would have been tested for HIV right at the start.

Because he did not fit their preconceptions none of the many doctors he consulted even thought to test him 'just in case'. I am sure they tested him for syphilis without asking his permission. It is standard practice - but test for HIV? Oh, no!

Perhaps, subconsciously, it would be threatening for most doctors to consider that a man of their own age, class and background could be 'at risk'. Perhaps it would call their own HIV status into question.

Whatever the reason, RT was allowed to suffer unnecessarily and, before he was given any treatment, his condition deteriorated to a point where he might die within days and improvement was unlikely.

But he did improve. Our wedding photos show a handsome, caring groom with no obvious sign of ill health. We were married at a tiny Registry Office with just my mother and her friend as witnesses. We then went to one of our favourite pubs for a celebratory meal and RT actually managed to eat a prawn cocktail, his first solid meal for months.

A confirmed and determined bachelor, RT had proposed out of a sense of duty. Now he suddenly discovered that he loved being married. I was his wife and for weeks he proudly boasted of this fact to anyone who would listen. Our relationship became deeper and closer. Our love was stronger than ever before.

CHAPTER 2

January 1995

By New Year's Day it was obvious that RT was not going to be dying immediately and we had to start learning how to live with AIDS.

What is it that makes AIDS such a nightmare? There are many other terminal diseases but, terrible though they are, none of them carry the stigma of HIV infection or create the same sort of panic as AIDS. It cannot be simply that AIDS is considered by some people to be self-inflicted. So are lung cancer and cirrhosis of the liver.

It may be that the uncharitable see AIDS as God's just retribution for unacceptable practices, but what about the children born HIV+, the haemophiliacs infected by their essential transfusions and blood products, the wives of closet bisexuals, the nurse who died because she stubbed her toe in a primitive, Third World operating theatre, and what about the people like RT who will never know how, when or why they became infected? RT felt as though he had become a modern leper who should be ringing a bell and crying, "Unclean! Unclean!" wherever he walked.

But it is the disease itself, not just the means of transmission, that is so frightening. It can lie dormant for years, unrecognised, quietly destroying the immune system, leaving the body vulnerable to innumerable, frequently simultaneous, opportunistic infections. With other terminal diseases the progression is usually well known. It may not be possible to predict how long the patient has to live or whether remission might occur but at least the symptoms can be described in advance and the treatments discussed.

With AIDS it is impossible to predict the course of the disease. A simple, common fungal infection like thrush may fail to respond to treatment and become a killer. Or the patient may develop cancer, tuberculosis, anaemia, chronic digestive problems, dementia, blindness, paralysis, pneumonia - or simply die of starvation because eating is too painful and nausea, drugs and depression have destroyed all appetite.

Frequently the symptoms are obvious but the cause is not. Many infections and drugs can create identical symptoms but will require different treatments for effective control. Several infections may attack at once, each one requiring different medication, some of it still experimental, so that the patient is taking dozens of pills to a complex timetable with increasing risks of unpleasant side-effects.

It is the unknown that terrifies and with AIDS so much is unknowable. Every new symptom could be the first sign of a new infection and may mean that the end is near. If the infection is identified it may respond to treatment but the new drugs might cause other problems. The threat of total disability, constant pain and nausea and a lingering death is ever present.

Added to all of this is the fear of rejection either by those who see the disease as proof of an unacceptable lifestyle, by those who fear infection or by loved ones who just cannot cope with all the suffering to come.

We had to decide what to tell people about RT's illness. There was no way he could accept any member of his family knowing the true diagnosis. He was sure they would think the worst (from his point of view) - that he was secretly bisexual or else injecting drugs. And who can blame him when even his doctor refused to discuss the source of his infection.

There are statistics that show how many cases of HIV infection have resulted so far from homosexual, bisexual, heterosexual, drugs or blood products transmission. But how are these figures compiled? No one would talk to RT about his infection. They dismissed his ideas of being infected in 1969 by blood transfusion as being impossible. They seemed to reject out of hand any thought of heterosexual transmission in the '70s. His doctor simply said, "A journalist? A man of the world? Travelled a lot? Ah well, we don't need to ask any more." The implication seemed to be that RT must have secrets that he would not wish to discuss in front of me.

By saying that "it doesn't matter how you were infected," the doctor was trying to appear non-judgemental but, for RT, it was a deep insult. It did matter to him how he became infected. It mattered to him that his doctor at least should believe him and be prepared to discuss the frightening implications. It mattered that he could never understand how he could possibly have this particular disease - it was a major cause of his ongoing depression, particularly as that hideous ulcer around his anus seemed, to him, to shout the false accusation, "Buggery!"

On the advice of our GP we decided to tell everyone that RT had leukaemia. The symptoms are very similar. Soon RT started to refer to his disease publicly as his 'Lucosade'. It was a sign that his sense of humour was returning and, I think, indicated that he would have liked to be able to talk openly about his illness rather than continuing to lie.

As the Christmas holidays finished we began to discover just what is meant by Care in the Community.

An Occupational Therapist, AC, was the first visitor. She came to assess RT's needs and co-ordinate the help we might need. Our tiny, sixteenth century cottage was really quite unsuitable for looking after an invalid but it was our home and we intended to stay there.

A new bath was a top priority. Ours was very small and deep, probably Victorian. It was too short for RT's bony, six-foot frame and the enamel had worn away leaving a surface that was rough, difficult to clean and very painful for his poor bottom. AC wanted us to switch to a walk-in shower but neither of us would contemplate doing without the comfort of a bath. RT needed a hot soak twice a day to ease the pains in his stiff joints and, for me, bathtime was the only opportunity I had to escape, to be by myself and relax.

Improvements to the kitchen were essential if I was to be able to maintain strict hygiene. Being 400 years old, the kitchen floor was just massive rough slabs of slate covered with some bitumen and ancient lino. It was so uneven that it was impossible to keep clean and I had never been able to have any fitted units at all.

Storage space was just a couple of old sideboards and the worktop was only 15 inches square. Spiders loved the gaping holes behind the beams and cobwebs appeared everywhere overnight.

AC contacted a charity that would help us with the applications for local authority grants for the work and would then deal with the builders on our behalf. She also decided to send a physiotherapist to help improve RT's mobility.

The physiotherapist was wonderful. She had considerable experience of the virus and was a natural counsellor who could really get RT to talk. She was the first person to give him any spark of hope. For her sake he would do his breathing exercises, go swimming and try the occasional press-up. He was very weak indeed and there was a lot of muscle wastage but he did make some improvement.

The second visit by the physiotherapist introduced us to another problem. She stood at the door and explained that she had a sore throat and so would not come in. She did not wish to risk giving RT another infection to cope with. Such a possibility had not yet occurred to us, but now we suddenly became aware of every cough and sneeze in the vicinity.

Our next therapist was the dietician. For a full week I had to keep a detailed diary of every mouthful of food and sip of liquid that passed RT's lips. This information was entered into a computer and an accurate assessment of his dietary needs calculated. She suggested stronger food supplements and provided various recipes to try to make them more palatable. They really did taste awful, just like synthetic milk-shakes, but RT persevered with them, forcing himself to drink two or three a day, and he did start to put on a little weight.

Then we were introduced to aromatherapy massage. For the first session I asked to be allowed to watch and learn. The therapist seemed surprised but reluctantly tolerated my presence and I carefully studied her movements and choice of oils. From then on, every night, I would massage RT until he relaxed enough to sleep.

A helpful Social Worker joined the stream of regular callers. This worried RT a little as he assumed that she was there just to make sure that he was not beating me up. On her first visit she arrived wearing strong make-up and bright red nail varnish. This scared RT and he immediately dubbed her Red Claws. On her second visit he refused to come downstairs to see her until she was just about to leave. She never again appeared with red nails and RT did soon learn to like and trust her - but the secret nickname stuck.

A homeopathist friend of mine, who had never met RT, talked to me at great length on the phone and prescribed some remedies for him. RT had little faith in alternative medicine but agreed to take the pills and I noticed an immediate, if slight, improvement in appetite and energy.

Amongst the mass of medication prescribed by his doctor, RT was taking a low dose of MST, the slow release version of morphine. Just the name morphine was enough to frighten him and he refused to take it twice a day as prescribed but agreed to have the evening dose because the night-time pains in his joints were preventing him from sleeping.

Its effect was dramatic. He would lie in bed quite happy but hallucinating. He would grab hold of my hand and try to change gear with it or try to smoke one of my fingers. He held invisible newspapers and struggled to turn the pages. He tried to open invisible drawers and cupboards. Occasionally he would get angry with something and lash out with his hands. If I was in the way I would get hit.

This behaviour would go on for much of the night and then he would sleep all day, getting up at 5pm to have a bath and go to the pub for an hour before trying to eat a small meal. But nausea and lack of appetite frustrated all his attempts to put back some weight. The doctor, while apologising for not being able to prescribe it, recommended cannabis as an excellent remedy for pain, nausea and stress. This took us completely by surprise. We had never contemplated using any recreational drugs other than alcohol and tobacco and wondered where to start.

Some discreet enquiries led us to a reliable local source both of the weed itself and advice on how to use it. I rolled some cigarettes and RT tried one. It had no effect, so he tried another - he was always impatient. Before I knew what he was up to he had smoked 5 joints and taken his morphine together with some brandy. He was high as a kite, happy and giggling. He ate very well that night.

After that we always had cannabis available but he didn't really like it very much. When he remembered he would use it to control the nausea and to help him relax but he preferred to rely on his old friend, alcohol. He decided not to take the MST any more. He did not enjoy sleeping every day away and would rather suffer some pain if necessary. For the first four days without morphine he felt very ill with stomach cramps and aching limbs. Then the pain eased and his sleeping patterns returned to normal.

Of course I was feeling stressed, confused, frightened and exhausted most of the time. My emotions seemed to be riding on a roller coaster, swooping sickeningly from low to high and back down again. The strangest feeling came just four days after the initial diagnosis. We still had no information other than that RT was HIV+ and were desperately worried. We had slept very little because RT was in great pain and I would be getting up two or three times a night to make him a cup of tea.

On the fourth day I suddenly felt extraordinarily happy - I think euphoric might be a better word for it. The sensation lasted for hours and seemed quite illogical. I can only assume that I had been under so much stress that my brain decided to release a 'happy' chemical to provide an artificial holiday from mental pain.

From then on I survived by keeping my brain busy. I did as much research into HIV and AIDS as was possible in such a rural area. I telephoned any relevant organisations I could track down and asked for whatever literature they could offer. One local advisory council proved really helpful and lent me books that, after buying my own copies, became essential sources of information on symptoms, infections, medication, side effects, alternative therapies, publications and much more. I set out to become an expert in my husband's illness so that, together, we could take back some control of our lives.

After the initial shock of reading about all the possible infections and side-effects that might occur at any time, I started to realise with some anger that every publication assumed that the patient would be homosexual. Heterosexuals were simply never mentioned.

The Gay Community has much to be proud of in its successful campaign to make the world aware of AIDS. It is thanks to the homosexuals that RT received such good treatment, care and financial assistance but every publication that he looked at or television programme that he watched reinforced his feeling that he had somehow contracted the 'Gay Plague' and had been 'put into the wrong box.'

RT admitted to being homophobic. When he was seventeen he had set off to hitch-hike round Europe. To his confusion and disgust every driver who picked him up immediately made sexual advances and then, when he refused them, threw him out of the car.

This happened many times over several days. He was young, innocent and frightened. He became convinced that this was normal, homosexual behaviour. He gave up, bought a train ticket and returned home.

Now, believing all the press reports, he understood that the 'Gay Plague' was in this country solely because of the activity of promiscuous homosexuals and he could not forgive them. Somehow they had infected him and anyone who learnt of his diagnosis must assume that he, too, was gay.

In our area there was just one respite centre, I shall call it The Convent, some twenty miles away. We were told that it was very good but might be too gay for us. I had no hope of getting RT to even look at the place.

But I knew that I needed respite and more support than I had found so far. When I happened to be passing I decided to drop in to The Convent to see what it was like. As I parked the car I found I was shaking and it was several minutes before I gathered the courage to walk to the door.

There was no sign of life. I rang the bell but no one came. The door was unlocked so I went in. There was silence and stillness. It had the appearance of a very smart and tastefully decorated guest house. There was a wonderful spicy smell of food cooking - but no people. I was too scared to go beyond the hallway and so I walked back to the car. In a way I was pleased that I would not have to tell RT about the visit. I was sure he would have been angry.

His temper had always been erratic and now, when he was feeling so ill and stressed, he had little tolerance for anything that was not exactly as he wished. He continued, most of the time, to present a charming face to the world. But in private he could not contain his rage.

He was aware that he was not coming to terms with his illness and started seeking for a source of spiritual guidance. He had a mental image of someone much older and wiser than he - perhaps a Jesuit with whom he could have philosophical discussions on the meaning of life and death. But such intellectuals are hard to find in the remote rural area in which we lived. Someone suggested that the manager of The Convent might have the right sort of contacts and an appointment was arranged for us to meet him.

With such a legitimate excuse it was just possible for RT to visit The Convent but he was still very disturbed by the idea. He was afraid that the place would be full of noisy, aggressive young homosexuals, all clad in black leather and wearing rings in their noses. In fact, on that day, the place again seemed deserted and we were not to meet any of the guests.

The Convent was created by a small group of nuns. They had realised the need for a respite centre in our area and succeeded in raising the money to convert a derelict building in the middle of their garden. The first impression on driving into the grounds is of a large attractive house in a private world of peace and quiet.

We were expected, greeted warmly, shown into a fairly large meeting room and offered tea which arrived on a beautifully presented tray with bone china crockery and some delicious cake. RT started to relax just a little.

The Manager arrived a few minutes later. He was considerably younger than us and had an almost ecclesiastical air about him. He was casually dressed but we did wonder if he was a monk in mufti. Our next thought was, "Perhaps he's gay."

Like most of the professionals we met at that time, he covered up his surprise at our appearance quite well but there was still a certain stiffness in his manner. He listened to our story but showed little response. He seemed to have some difficulty at first in understanding just what sort of spiritual advisor RT was looking for. Eventually he thought he knew exactly the right person, the chaplain at the local university, and he offered to arrange a meeting whenever RT was ready. He then showed us around the house and explained that we were welcome to stay there when we needed some respite.

The house was certainly beautiful. The main room was vast with windows on three sides looking out over the attractive gardens. The decoration was tasteful and peaceful. The furniture comfortable and inviting. There was an atmosphere of calm.

The bedrooms seemed large, well decorated and very clean. Some were double, some single. Each one had an en-suite shower or bath and a small kitchen nearby for nocturnal refreshments. A conservatory had been built to provide a pleasant smoking room and the tiny Quiet Room had a dramatic stained glass window that had been specially designed to encourage thoughts of hope and spiritual uplift in those with HIV, their carers and the bereaved.

The Convent seemed to be somewhere where we might find some peace - but what about the other guests? We had yet to meet any and did not know what they might be like. As we left I wondered if RT would allow us to return there soon. I thought probably not.

One question cropped up again and again. What was my HIV status? Had I been infected?

The first to ask was our GP. He was fairly insistent that I should be tested straight away. When I hesitated he said to RT, "She doesn't want it because she thinks she might be infected." He seemed to be worried that I might go around infecting other men. The more he pushed me the more I became convinced that now was not the time for testing.

I was, and still am, feeling very healthy. The chances of infection were slight but, of course, it was a possibility. I felt that, if I were tested now, whatever the result, it would be damaging for RT. If I were in the clear then he would feel even more isolated, even more a pariah. If I were infected then he would feel guilty.

So I chose to wait. I would not be tested until some symptoms occurred or RT died.

CHAPTER 3

Spring 1995

"You have taken up your bed and walked!" enthused the doctor. He could hardly believe the improvement in RT's health He was certainly much stronger and more mobile. He could now do a very few press-ups, was breathing better and swimming four widths of our small local pool nearly every day. The physiotherapist decided that he no longer needed her help and said, "Goodbye."

But he didn't feel well. His bottom and nose had both healed completely and his mouth was much less painful but still he felt ill, exhausted and depressed. Every night he was being woken up by an agonising pain in his chest. He described it as a steamroller just sitting on him and nothing seemed to help. The doctor treated it as an ulcer and prescribed Zantac to be added to the steadily increasing number of pills that RT was swallowing every day. I made sure that he changed from aspirin to paracetamol for his routine painkillers - just in case his stomach lining was damaged. But there was no improvement.

He was no longer suffering so much pain in his joints at night because the Community Care nurse had arrived bearing a special pressure relieving mattress that made all the difference. It made a difference to me too. We shared a double bed. This new mattress was very thick and at least three foot wide. It occupied two thirds of the bed leaving only an eighteen inch strip for me.

Perhaps it was the added stress of trying to sleep while clinging on to the edge of the bed, or perhaps it was just that, with RT starting to improve, I now felt free to fall apart - for some reason I seemed less able to cope than before. I was deeply tired.

The change in me must have been obvious because RT raised no objection when I suggested that we book into The Convent for a week. Red Claws would arrange the finances from the Social Services budget so I just had to ring the manager and set a date.

We had three weeks to wait before our visit. I had three weeks more of trying to cope with our shattered lives before I could rest. Then fate threw us another blow.

The cottage is built into the side of a hill. The road runs past at roof level and there are fields beyond it. All the rainwater from the road and fields flows down into a gully just outside the kitchen door where a drain carries it away, under the kitchen and out to the sewers.

One night, when RT's pain woke us as usual for our 3am cup of tea, we discovered that there was a blackout. I lit a candle and went downstairs to see if the old-fashioned mains trip-switch had been triggered by a thunderstorm. As I stepped off the bottom of the stairs my foot sank into two inches of water. The entire ground floor was flooded. I found a torch and peered out through the kitchen window. It was pouring with rain. The gully was overflowing and water was seeping under the kitchen door. There was nothing I could do in the dark so I went back to bed.

As soon as it was daylight I asked my mother to come and help and together we commenced mopping up. RT had not understood when I told him that we were flooded. He was angry that I was not beside him when he woke. He stormed off to have a bath shouting for me to bring him coffee, refusing to listen to any explanations of why I couldn't look after him at the moment.

When he finally came downstairs and saw what had happened, he went straight back to bed. This was more than he could handle and it was an affront to his masculinity that my mother and I had been left to cope with a crisis that, in healthier days, he would have dealt with himself.

He later apologised for his behaviour but he was simply not strong enough to help us to carry the wet carpets out to the greenhouse where they could be left to drip themselves dry.

I checked the drain and found that it was not blocked. It must have been an exceptionally heavy downpour. The carpets slowly dried and my mother helped me to set everything to rights.

It was such a relief to be setting off for The Convent at last. Over the past few days I had been able to sense a change in myself as though, after four months, I was just beginning to come out of a state of shock that had been protecting me from the full realisation of the frightening and uncertain future that we faced. I now needed to talk to other people who, already having some experience and knowledge of the disease, could understand the confusion and pain I was experiencing.

Of course we arrived full of tension and fear. We knew that the building was comfortable and very pleasant, with an air of solidity, stability and peace, but what of our fellow guests? How would we cope? Would there be any other guests from our area who might recognise us and disclose our terrible secret to our neighbours?

We were welcomed by a Sister who gave us the surprising news that the Manager had left his post the previous week. This certainly added to my tension, as did the Sister's obvious surprise at the kind of people we were. She clearly thought we might not fit in, and our fear of our fellow guests increased. The atmosphere in the building was one of confusion, a time of change and uncertainty.

The Manager had told us to arrive in time for lunch but we now felt that this was too early and we were in the way. It was change-over day, our room was not yet ready and everyone was far too busy to spend time making us feel at home.

Our double room proved reassuring. It was comfortably large with two windows so that we could ensure a good flow of air. RT needed cold, fresh air to help his breathing. But there was a shower rather than a bath. RT panicked at the thought of being deprived of his regular, muscle-easing soak. I explained our problem to the Sister who immediately solved it by finding us a bath elsewhere in the building that we could use.

After a long siesta we dashed out to the pub to build up the courage to meet our fellow guests over dinner. RT insisted that he would not, under any circumstances, be swapping symptoms over the dinner table.

Everyone looked surprisingly normal and the food was delicious. We found ourselves sitting opposite an ex-teacher, J, who proved to be a regular visitor and long-term survivor who had helped in the original renovation of the house. His gentle, intelligent manner disarmed RT who, despite his earlier protestations, was soon telling his story and asking questions about the disease. I was so pleased to see him opening up and relaxing. For the first time he was really talking about HIV and how it was affecting his life.

Getting acquainted with the other guests took a bit longer. The next day we found ourselves trapped in the Conservatory with two rather drunken Irishmen discussing their religious differences. We made our escape and went out for a walk to a nearby National Trust property. At this time of year the gardens were open free of charge and we enjoyed an unexpectedly sunny interlude amongst the beautiful magnolias. RT walked much further than we expected.

Over dinner we talked again with J and then went straight to our room. This meant that we missed all the excitement. The Irishmen, who had been drinking continuously since they arrived, had become abusive. They were attacking the other guests, mostly verbally I think, and causing considerable upset to people who, like ourselves, had come to The Convent for some essential respite. The staff called in reinforcements and the troublesome pair were escorted to the station and put on a train for home.

The incident was the talk of the breakfast table next morning and it really broke the ice. RT found he was able to chat and laugh with his fellow guests despite his concerns about their sexuality.

The atmosphere at The Convent encouraged relaxation. There was plenty of space to move freely - very important for someone like RT whose stiff limbs made him clumsy at times. The rooms had been arranged to provide quiet areas for intimate conversations or solitude. The gardens were attractive even in the early spring. And, most important for us, the food was inviting, tempting RT to eat much more than before.

I was able to sleep, read and eat without worrying about the housekeeping, cooking or shopping. I could devote much more of my time to keeping RT company or else seize the opportunity to escape by myself for a while, knowing that he would be well looked after.

Our only problem was with smoking. Out of fourteen guests I was the only non-smoker. Most of the staff smoked too. But smoking was not allowed anywhere except in the Conservatory and the Smokers' Lobby.

The Smokers' Lobby was tiny and, with a stone floor and stone-clad walls, seemed designed to give the impression that smokers were banished from the house. In fact the Lobby itself has now become a smoke-free zone because it is too near the kitchen.

The Conservatory provided a pleasant alternative but it was sometimes very crowded and thick with smoke - quite unsuitable for quiet contemplation or a private conversation and, being at the end of a long corridor, you could not tell who was in there until it was too late to retreat without seeming rude.

RT's doctor had told him not to try to cut down on cigarettes as that would increase his stress and aggravate his breathing difficulties. I imagine that it was the same for many of the guests and that, like RT, they found that those lonely sleepless hours of fear and pain in the middle of the night are just when a cigarette can be vital medicine.

In our room we kept the windows wide open and RT smoked when he needed to, despite the regulations. We were very careful not to set off the smoke alarm and no one complained.

Before he left, the Manager had arranged for his friend, the Chaplain at the university, to visit RT while he was staying at The Convent. RT was pleased to have a chance to meet him. Before the illness had made him too weak, RT had started on the preliminary research for his Ph.D. at the university. He hoped the Chaplain, as well as being his spiritual adviser, might be able to give him some guidance on whether it would be possible to continue his studies on a part-time basis if his strength continued to improve.

The occasion was not a success. It was clear from the moment he entered that the Chaplain, Father B, was not the sort of person RT needed. He was too young, too casually dressed (no dog-collar) and fairly obviously gay. He had great difficulty understanding what sort of spiritual help RT might need. He was a bit more constructive about the possibilities of returning to study part-time and told us that there were already a couple of students known to be HIV+ who were well accepted.

But Father B obviously found RT very difficult to understand. His sense of humour was too dry, his questions too intellectually demanding and his homophobia too obvious. The Chaplain terminated the discussion as quickly as possible and talked to the other guests leaving RT feeling rejected and hurt. He promised to visit us at home but we never heard from Father B again except for a brief postcard promising to see us soon.

RT had brought his own occupational therapy with him. He had recently developed a passion for polishing wood, any sort of wood, and on our earlier visit he had noticed the ornate banisters and carved newel posts on The Convent's staircase. So he brought cleaners and polishes in his suitcase and spent much of the first few days slowly working his way up the stairs. It made him feel that he was contributing something to this wonderful place.

He was looking much better and enjoying his stay. I had found in a local greengrocer's some Chilean strawberries. This was only the first week of March but these strawberries were large, delicious and cheap. RT asked me to buy enough strawberries and cream to provide a treat for everyone at The Convent. I bought far too many.

The huge bowl was brought in at lunchtime and everyone cheered - the surprise was a great success. There were more strawberries than we could eat and the leftovers went into a flan and a massive strawberry cake as well as providing the essential ingredient for a strawberry and yoghurt fool.

Despite all the rest, good food and friendly people, I still felt anxious. I knew that I needed to talk. I had hoped that on the very first day someone would sit down with me and ask me what I needed to get out of the week - but no one did. I was the only female guest and I felt very alone, particularly in the afternoons when RT was asleep. I would sit for hours in the sitting room, hoping that someone would come and talk - but I was always left to myself. I tried going into the Smokers' Lobby and the Conservatory, but they were noisy and crowded - I just couldn't cope.

Towards the end of the week I knew that I would have to send out louder signals for help, though I was not sure how. Once again I was sitting alone. I had wandered around the gardens in the sleet; sat in the potting shed and cried; retreated from the crowded Lobby and returned to the sitting room. But that was soon invaded by a noisy trio seeking music.

By now the Lobby was empty, so I sat there. The member of staff on duty, B, noticed my solitude and came to offer companionship and a friendly ear. She was a great help.

Perhaps she spoke to V who was on the night shift - I don't know. Anyway, later that evening, V extracted me from the crowded Lobby on the pretext of helping her to make some coffee. She sat me down at the kitchen table and encouraged me to talk. We were there until way past bedtime and my depression started to lift.

The next day it was time to go home. Much to RT's surprise all the other guests insisted on hugging and kissing him goodbye. They had accepted him completely and forgave his homophobia. He responded well, though with a certain embarrassment.

As we left the staff reminded us that we were welcome to come back at any time. We could use The Convent as a day centre if we wished and just had to give them a ring if we wanted a meal or the alternative therapies. We promised to return soon.

We were both stronger and calmer for our week of respite, but it was good to be home again. RT was still being woken by his steamroller every night. Sometimes he was crying with the pain for two hours before the pain killers would take effect. He stopped taking the Zantac as it was obviously not helping.

He believed he would die before the end of the year. With a CD4 cell count of only 20 he was sure that his case was hopeless and, with the ongoing pain in his muscles and joints and his digestion problems, the depression and exhaustion just got deeper.

All the published information on AIDS seemed to deal with cases with CD4 cell counts of over 200. Anything lower was hardly mentioned and this reinforced RT's conviction that he could not possibly feel any better. He was often impatient to get the dying over and done with.

But he persevered with the swimming and tried to learn how to relax and improve his posture to relieve some of the physical causes of stress. He forced himself to eat and to take the homeopathic remedies. He started seeing a chiropractor in case he could ease some of the pain - but RT found the treatment itself too rough and soon stopped. We decided, with the doctor's agreement, to stop taking the prophylactic antibiotic as there was no sign of any chest infection and the antibiotic itself could well be making him feel ill. I kept a supply of the antibiotic in the cupboard so that at the first sign of any chest problems I could give him the medication before calling out the doctor.

I had been keeping a diary since the diagnosis and I now encouraged him to read it so that he could see that, even though he still felt very ill indeed, he had improved greatly over the past weeks.

What he needed most was some encouragement from his doctor to believe that further improvement was possible and that he wasn't necessarily facing a future of unremitting pain, exhaustion and nausea. But his doctor believed in straight talking and not offering any false hopes. He simply insisted on reminding RT that the virus would kill him and that he had already improved more than had been expected - no wonder his depression deepened.

To relieve the depression he increased his consumption of brandy. Sometimes it worked and we could spend a pleasant evening together - but then he would have just one more and his mood would turn to anger. At such times he could become very aggressive, negative and hurtful. He needed me to be unnaturally strong. I mustn't show any pain, tiredness or distress because he couldn't cope with it. He was the one who was ill and he considered it my job as his wife to look after him with a constant smile no matter what he said or did.

He was being totally unreasonable. I fought back, argued, cried, shouted and even hit out - but in the end, because I knew how desperate was his need for love and understood the mental and physical torture he was suffering, I always forgave.

Many times he apologised for his behaviour and thanked me for staying with him. We needed each other and our love was strong.

One evening, when he was feeling rather maudlin, he rang his mother. They did not get on well together and he had not yet told her about his illness. Suddenly, much to his surprise, he found himself telling her that he had leukaemia and would probably die very soon. He then handed the telephone to me so that I could explain. She took the news calmly. From her experience dying young was what most men did. Her second husband had died from leukaemia at the age of forty-seven.

I told her that treatments had much improved since those days and reassured her that, while RT's condition might deteriorate at any time, there was a good chance that he would respond to the drugs and enjoy a period of remission. This seemed to satisfy her and I was able to say goodnight and turn my attention to RT who had frightened himself with this unplanned conversation. He couldn't eat at all. His night was punctuated with bad dreams and several times I woke to find him crying in his sleep.

The next evening his mother rang to say that she had bought a large medical dictionary and could I please explain to her just what sort of leukaemia RT had and what treatment he was receiving. She couldn't understand why a bone marrow transplant wasn't being considered.

We had a similar problem with a friend who, on being told that RT was suffering from leukaemia, informed us that her sister-in-law's brother was the top specialist in leukaemia and that she would arrange an appointment for us to see him immediately.

I hated all this lying. I could understand RT's need for secrecy but it was adding to our stress.

We were, at this time, waiting for the results of RT's second CD4 cell count. He had improved so much over the past few months that he was sure the number would have increased. A brief letter came from the doctor saying, "All your blood test results show you are maintaining Status Quo. We won't talk about the CD4 count."

RT refused to show any emotion. He simply dictated a reply for me to dispatch by return of post. It read, "Message received and understood. Who's counting anyway?" That stiff upper lip again. He was devastated by the news.

He started sleeping round the clock once more. He would panic at the thought of food and would have to lie down immediately after eating anything to try to control the nausea. The pains in his chest increased and he was worried about his lungs. His mouth became sore and dry again - the candida was back. His guts started churning and rumbling all day long. Athletes' foot attacked his toes making walking very painful. He became obsessed with his weight, weighing himself at least twice a day. The steamroller pain returned every night and could only be eased by cuddling an electric hot-pad, drinking hot tea and having his head massaged.

It was more than a month since we had left The Convent and RT refused to go back for a visit. He threw himself into his gardening. He would drive himself to exhaustion, cutting the grass and hedges, pruning bushes, creating new flower beds, spreading compost and planting dahlias, runner beans, strawberries and, of course, our own tiny, secret patch of cannabis.

It was the garden that helped him then. The weather was good and when he was tired he could just sit and enjoy the view that he loved, down the valley and out to sea. And he did get very tired. He could work for no more than a few minutes before collapsing in a chair, but he wouldn't give up and slowly he became a little stronger and calmer.

The time had come for a dental check-up. This worried him. Should he tell the dentist of his infection? Would the receptionist be discreet? He agreed with me that it was essential that the dentist should know everything as there might be some special treatment that he could offer. But what if the dentist rejected him? That was a situation RT could not bear to contemplate.

At last he allowed me to visit the dentist alone to explain the situation. The dentist was most understanding and sympathetic. There was no question at all of refusing to treat RT and, in fact, he gave him preferential treatment, working very slowly, gently and carefully, explaining everything that he did but never mentioning the diagnosis in the presence of his assistant or writing it down on the notes.

As the weather got warmer so RT gained in strength. He seemed to be finding some pleasure in life again and learning to cope with his disabilities. He was eating better, putting on weight, walking further, cracking jokes and having a little fun. But then it was time for another visit to the clinic.

He always got very worked up before an appointment, would drink too much, refuse to eat and become noticeably anxious. But this particular meeting went well. After lunch I left him at the hospital for his aromatherapy massage session and drove to the nearby shops. Suddenly, at a very busy and dangerous junction, the car made horrific grinding noises and stopped dead.

Fortunately there was a pub nearby and I was able to ring the hospital and the rescue services who were absolutely marvellous. I explained my problem and they had a relay truck at the scene within ten minutes. The car was put on board and we were taken to the hospital to pick up RT - only five minutes late!

I knew what the problem was. A c.v. joint had collapsed for the third time in two years, which suggested that perhaps the chassis was out of alignment. Maybe the car had been in a serious accident before we bought it. Whatever the reason - it was clearly time to get rid of this car. What if it had broken down, miles from anywhere, while RT was on board? Neither of us could cope with the stress of continually listening for strange noises, wondering if they were symptoms of yet more trouble. We needed a good, reliable car - one with power steering so that RT could start to drive again, and one with enough room to carry a wheelchair in case RT should need one in the future.

Unfortunately Income Support does not stretch far enough for such luxuries. We had no savings and could not afford to borrow enough for the sort of car we needed. We considered using RT's Mobility Allowance to lease a car from Motability but discovered that when he died the car would be instantly repossessed unless I could find the cash to buy it outright. So I would be left without a car just at the time when I would be emotionally unable to deal with any extra problems.

Finally I remembered that there were several charities related to my profession. I chose one at random and rang the secretary. She was most sympathetic and sure that they would be able to help. I wrote a long letter and filled in their application form. A few weeks later came the reply offering me £1000 towards the car and also offering to forward my application to two other charities who might be able to give us some further assistance. Of course I readily agreed. It looked like we would soon have our new car.

This generous response from the charity triggered a gradual change in RT's perception of the world. That he might receive financial help from people who had never met him was an astounding idea. Slowly he came to understand that there are good people around - he had just not met very many so far or else failed to recognise their attributes. He had always had a completely cynical view of mankind but now he was just beginning to discover that some people might be worthy of his friendship and trust.

I was still riding that emotional roller-coaster. Understandably my mood usually reflected RT's state of health and that could change several times a day.

The constant stream of Care in the Community visitors had ceased. The hospital appointments were now at 6 week intervals and Red Claws came to see us once a month - and that was it. The rest of the time we were on our own in a remote rural community where only my mother and the GP knew of RT's true diagnosis.

There were some good times, times of sunshine and laughter, times of sharing and affection, times of peace, times of sensible and serious conversation. But there were also many times of fear, anger and anxiety. RT wanted to know what was going to happen to him. All his current symptoms could be caused by the depression or the medication - or were they symptoms typical of late HIV infection? The books were of no help. They talked about opportunistic infections but made no mention of the likely progress of the disease when all the infections were under control. Nowhere could I find a book that explained what it might be like to die of AIDS.

In times of despair, when RT longed to die, we talked for hours about our respective beliefs in life after death. We shared what little we knew about dying. RT dreaded the thought of more pain - he had suffered so much already. But what frightened him most was the Death Certificate. Would it say he died of AIDS? So many people need to see the Death Certificate - his family might see it - it might be mentioned in the newspapers - ...

I promised to do everything I could to keep his secret from his family and we agreed to ask the doctor about Death Certificates at our next visit.

Soon after our return from The Convent there had been a heavy rainstorm and water again flooded under the backdoor. This time I saw it happen and managed to get most of the carpets up and furniture moved before too much damage was done - but there was obviously something wrong with the drain.

We still had our tiny, battered, Victorian bathtub and the unhygienic kitchen. There had been little progress on the grant application, but, eventually, the man from the Council came round to make his assessment. I mentioned the flooding but he was not impressed. He told me that he only had my word for it that any water came in and obviously thought that I was trying to cheat the system somehow.

A couple of weeks later I came down one morning to find the living room flooded again. I rang the man from the Council and asked him to come and help with the mopping up. He arrived within the hour but didn't try to help. He did, however, agree that there was a problem with the drain.

The slow wheels of bureaucracy started to turn and I had hopes that we might soon have a decent bath, a real kitchen and dry carpets. But then, I always was an optimist.

As RT regained a little strength and began to discuss the possibility of attempting to work for his Ph.D. again, I started to make some long-term plans for my future. I had applied for training for some freelance work that I would really enjoy and that, as long as I was good at it, I would be able to continue well into my seventies. The training involved spending the occasional day in London.

After my first trip RT confessed that he had really not been able to cope at all well without me. He had become dizzy and confused, unable to eat anything and more depressed and morbid than ever. He had forgotten to take his medication and refused my mother's offers of help.

I didn't know what to do. This training was important to me. I needed the security of knowing that I could be sure of being able to earn a living if RT died. I would have to be in London for two days in the early summer - how would RT manage? Could I leave him?

RT surprised me. He decided that he would come to London with me. We would drive up and stay with his mother. This positive plan seemed to stimulate his strength. He became more active and some days we were able to drive out to favourite locations for lunch and a walk.

On one of these outings we happened to pass near The Convent. I said nothing but, as we came up to the junction he told me to take the Convent road as he wanted to stop there for a cup of tea. I could sense his tension as we drove in.

Before I could park the car several members of staff came rushing out, all smiles, to greet us. They hugged RT warmly and made us feel so welcome that it was like coming home. RT asked if he could come back for a massage the following week. They said why not come for lunch too and booked me in for some reflexology.

I was so relieved. Here were people who understood what we were going through. These were friends we could trust. We were no longer so alone.

CHAPTER 4

Summer 1995

It was time to set off for London. We had borrowed my mother's car for the trip. It was older than ours but bigger, more reliable, more comfortable and, most importantly, it had power steering and RT would be able to do some of the driving.

RT had woken feeling very rough. He couldn't eat any breakfast. He started to cough and that triggered a bout of vomiting. The thought of the long drive and then staying with his mother for two days terrified him, but he was determined to go.

Despite feeling so poorly, RT decided to take the first shift as driver. His driving was a little erratic to start with - it had been so long since he had been strong enough to take the wheel of our small but heavy car - however, he soon found his rhythm again and was enjoying being back in control. He drove for three hours before exhaustion forced him to stop.

We stuck to the scenic route, avoiding the motorway and all the heavy traffic. It was a road he knew well with many favourite pubs, villages, cathedrals and walks on the way. So we took our time, enjoying the scenery and stopping for a rest whenever the mood took us. We visited a cathedral, walked on the hills and explored the architecture of some ancient villages. It was a wonderful day.

The nearer we got to London, however, the more tense he got. We stopped at a pub that had, for many years, been one of his regular haunts. We strolled along the banks of the trout stream that ran past the gardens and fed the last of our sandwiches to the greedy ducks before going inside for a drink. He was clearly reluctant to go on to his mother's house. Eventually he explained that whenever he had taken one of his girlfriends home there had always been arguments and he was afraid that I would quarrel with her.

I had only met her once, some years before. We had spoken many times on the telephone and, since the wedding, she had obviously accepted me fully as one of the family. I was able to reassure RT that, no matter what happened or was said, I would not quarrel with his mother.

We finally arrived at her home about an hour late. She proved to be elderly, independent, dogmatic and very set in her ways. Her health was not good but she was coping with life and enjoying her new, tiny flat right next to the shops. She and RT really did not understand each other at all and neither was prepared to make the effort to see the other's point of view but, for my sake, both took great pains to be polite and keep the peace.

Having been most concerned to find out what RT now liked to eat, his mother had generously bought in special supplies and presented us with a remarkable meal of King Prawns followed by smoked chicken, boiled potatoes and cabbage. It was delicious, if a little rich for RT's delicate digestion, and we both ate well. But we had the same menu again the next day, and the following day and again as a packed lunch for our journey home. I'm afraid that, by this time, smoked chicken had lost its appeal.

After the long journey and the strain of enforced politeness, RT slept well. The next day was a Sunday and he felt strong enough to drive me into the centre of London for my appointment. He spent the rest of the day exploring his old haunts in the City. When he picked me up in the evening he was in an excellent mood. The City had been absolutely deserted. He had wandered the empty streets remembering his early career and looking at the buildings that, when he started out in Chartered Surveying, had been the focus of his work.

Before returning to his mother's flat he took a detour to Chelsea to show me the scenes of his earlier, bachelor years and to tell me stories of that time of luxurious flats, fast cars and beautiful models. We were late for our prawns and smoked chicken but his good mood lasted and he was able to chat happily with his mother for hours.

The Monday he spent re-exploring the Downs. Later I joined him at Hampton Court where he showed me round the gardens that he had loved so much in his youth. He was strong, bright, charming and affectionate. These two days of solitary freedom, driving where he wished and recalling happier days, had done him so much good.

That evening I met, for the first time, his brother, sister-in-law and tiny niece. RT had the task of explaining about his 'leukaemia'. It was, inevitably, a shock for them. I still found the lying hard to handle and kept out of the conversation as much as possible.

Saying goodbye to his mother the next morning was difficult. He was convinced that he would never see her again. She had been brought up not to show emotion and their farewells were stiff and formal. RT was deeply depressed.

He again decided to drive the first leg of the journey and slowly his mood lifted as we took a meandering route down country lanes that held so many memories for him.

With the encouraging success of this journey behind him, RT's mood became more positive. He was eager to go to The Convent each week, forced himself to swim most days, worked hard in the garden and managed to eat a reasonable amount of food. His weight started to go up.

He was certainly feeling better but when I came to write out his list of current symptoms for the next appointment with his doctor I realised just how much pain he was fighting. At all times there was the chronic fatigue, both mental and physical. His muscles were very weak and the weight of his head made his neck ache. All his joints, but especially the knees and hips, ached continuously and would keep him awake at night. He was losing all sensation in his left foot and it had become very cold. (His right foot had been numb, cold and rigid ever since that appalling car crash so many years ago.) He was becoming very clumsy and seemed to be losing his sense of balance. There were dizzy spells, continuous, exhausting hiccups, nausea all the time, headaches, pains in the chest, massive coughing fits, gut ache and that frightening steamroller at night. Sometimes his nose would bleed. His mouth was itching and the sores at the corners of his lips had returned. Unsurprisingly he was showing signs of great anxiety and stress.

The doctor was not much help. He seemed not to hear the desperation in RT's voice and told him that he was lucky to be alive, could die at any time, would probably never feel any better and that his CD4 count had dropped to just 12. The doctor could offer no real hope of keeping the word AIDS off the Death Certificate as the authorities in our area had set very strict guidelines. The final blow of the meeting came when he revealed that the latest tests had shown a high level of Cytomegalovirus (CMV) in RT's blood. He could not tell whether the CMV was active or not but considered it important to start treating it just in case it was the cause of the current symptoms.

RT was devastated. On the way home he drank far too much brandy and became abusive and argumentative. The next day he felt absolutely awful. He was doubled up with stomach cramps. I managed to get him to The Convent where a massage just knocked him out. He was exhausted and emotional but the company of the sympathetic staff and volunteers did help him to lift his spirits just a little.

As he didn't ask, I didn't discuss the implications of the CMV. I knew only too well that this was the one infection he would fear beyond all others. It could progress very rapidly to leave him blind, demented, paralysed and incontinent. The treatment was experimental and the long list of possible side-effects too terrible to contemplate. There was only one piece of good luck - the medication was now available in capsules which could be swallowed, twelve of them each day. Until very recently the only treatment had been by intravenous infusion which would have meant being attached to a drip for at least an hour two or three times every day for the rest of his life. If RT did not know about CMV and did not want to ask, then I was certainly not going to tell him.

Slowly he regained some of his positive attitude and his strength improved. He managed to swim 18 widths one day when we had the pool to ourselves. He felt the need to get out, away from the cottage. Whenever the weather was fine we would drive out to find quiet pubs, beautiful scenery and to look at cars.

I had heard nothing from the charity for some weeks. There was no reply when I telephoned so I decided to contact the secretary of one of the other charities to see if my application had been forwarded as promised. She knew nothing about it and my heart sank. As I had to go up to London again the next day, she asked me to drop in to see her.

I was with her for about an hour and left her office in a daze, unable to believe what she had told me. I had explained our problem, giving her a copy of the original application. Her response was immediate. She could not speak for her directors but she was sure they would want to help with the car and that she could get other charities to join in. In fact she rang one of them on the spot to get a verbal assurance that they would be prepared to help. She then arranged for an instant emergency grant of £500 from her funds to help cover our current living expenses. She also told me that her directors would probably offer me a small monthly grant that would be disregarded by Social Security and so not affect our Income Support payments. They would also be quite likely to offer some help with meeting domestic bills.

Such overwhelming generosity was completely unexpected. My emotions were already battered. In my exhausted state I wandered the streets trying to make sense of the meeting. I needed to talk to someone so I dragged a friend from her office. We went for a coffee while I tried to explain what had happened but words were inadequate. There was just no way that I could express the complexity of emotions that were flooding through me.

I did little work that day. I was eager to rush home, tell RT the good news and start looking at cars in earnest.

RT's moods were fluctuating wildly. There were times when he would feel almost happy. Then suddenly anxiety would set in, he would feel trapped and frightened. He was terrified that he might need to go into hospital - would he ever get out again? More and more the brandy would push him into anger. He had wild fantasies of undertaking some great suicide mission, dying in a blaze of glory. He dreamt of adopting a little boy and being the perfect father for the short time he might have left. He fretted about his Ph.D. which he saw as his one chance to prove to the world that he had something worthwhile to contribute.

Sometimes he could hardly find the strength of will to get out of bed. Other days he would throw himself into manic activity in the garden, forcing himself to carry on past the point of exhaustion.

The hiccups were getting worse. At times he was feverish and frequently talked in his sleep. He had developed a slight tremor that was worrying but also had its funny side. He would lie in bed laughing as he watched his penis shaking uncontrollably as though it had life of its own.

When we returned to the clinic his doctor at last understood the depth of RT'S depression and anxiety. He realised that we had been left to cope on our own for far too long. Suddenly the tiny consulting room was full of nurses and health advisers offering suggestions on the way forward. The Community Nurse would now visit us at home regularly. The Macmillan Service would be notified so that one of their nurses could also visit us frequently. A 'Buddy' would be sought as a companion to provide us with ongoing friendship and help. An informal meeting would be arranged with the Chest Specialist who would be responsible for RT if he needed to be admitted to hospital.

It was all too much for RT. He was confused and his face looked grey. After a massage he was so drained he could hardly walk back to the car. That evening he managed to force himself to eat a few fish fingers and chips before collapsing into bed.

The next morning he was feverish and vomiting. He was continually straining to pass urine but his bladder was empty. He seemed to me to be dehydrated. I rang the clinic and arranged for the doctor to talk to our GP who rushed over to see us. It was a urine infection - one of the known side-effects of that experimental drug.

RT's temperature continued to rise. When he was awake he was coughing and vomiting all the time. Then he became delirious and we had a very disturbed night. By the morning I could see some improvement. The antibiotic was starting to work. He was drinking water and managed to eat some tinned peach slices. He was still coughing which triggered a fairly heavy nose bleed. Then he went back to sleep, sweating profusely.

The GP arrived unexpectedly to check up on his patient. Not allowing me time to wake RT, he dashed up the stairs so that RT woke suddenly, soaking wet and in a state of confusion. He started coughing and the GP, noticing the bloody tissues in the bin, assumed the worst. He wanted to call an ambulance but RT refused to go to hospital, so reluctantly the GP agreed to wait another 24 hours before making a decision.

He then led me down stairs where he told me that there was no point in forcing RT to go into hospital. He recognised the signs and knew that RT would die within the next two days. We might as well let him die in peace, at home.

Fortunately I did not believe him. A few hours later RT's temperature dropped. He got up, had a bath and insisted on being taken to the pub. He only managed a few mouthfuls of beer which, as soon as we got home, he vomited back up. But he had made his point. He was not ready to give up yet.

By the next day he was much improved though very weak. He was most concerned that the GP had thought he was dying. Suddenly the possibility of death became very real to him. He now asked me about CMV and I read him the relevant sections from the medical books. He was frightened at first but then seemed to become calmer, happier and more relaxed. He slept well that night. So did I. The Community Care Nurse had brought us a new mattress - a double one so that I could be comfortable too.

The improvement continued. Feeling and warmth had started to return to his left foot. The bed was no longer being drenched with sweat. After a week he found that beer was tasting good again. He was able to swim and play pool. There was a definite sense of pride in having overcome his first major opportunistic infection.

The Test Match at Lord's was starting in a few days. Would RT be strong enough to attend? It was an occasion that he never missed and we were determined that he should be there.

He was continuing to make a good recovery from the urine infection. All the old, familiar symptoms were still there and he was now complaining of a feeling like "rats gnawing in the belly" at night. But he was eating reasonably well and felt no worse than on the earlier trip to London.

So, having packed a large bag with all the medication necessary for a whole week away from home, we set off in my mother's car once again. And, once again, he was able to drive for the first three hours. It was not such a happy journey this time. RT was feeling uncomfortable and started drinking at lunchtime. I think he was worrying about spending five days at Lord's.

His membership of the M.C.C. was important to him. When attending matches he had always made a point of dressing immaculately and walking straight and tall, like a Guards Officer, even when he was feeling a great deal of pain, as he so often was. His leg had been so badly damaged in that awful car crash that the doctors told him he would never walk properly again. He proved them wrong but the knee and hip ached most of the time. Yet his pride would not allow him to be seen by fellow M.C.C. members with anything but a good British stiff upper lip and military bearing.

This time he knew he would not be able to hide his illness. RT could not walk without a stick. Those who knew him would be bound to notice his loss of weight and the deep lines that continuous pain had etched into his face. And I could not be with him. Women are still not allowed in the Pavilion during matches. He did not know if he could cope without me.

He drove into St John's Wood through the London weekday traffic and succeeded eventually in finding a Disabled Parking space - the only one in the area, half a mile from the cricket ground. Apparently the day went well but he was grey with exhaustion when I met him at the gates at the end of play.

RT was still tired and tense as he drove off the next morning. When I met him later there had been a transformation. He was relaxed, drunk and happy despite having got a Parking Ticket for overstaying his welcome on the Disabled Meter.

That morning, as he had slowly walked into the Long Room, a stranger, JK, who was also visibly disabled, had greeted RT with great fellow feeling and invited him for a drink. Their friendship deepened as the day progressed.

The next day was Saturday, always an important social occasion at the Test Match, and JK was fulfilling a long-held and very expensive ambition. He had succeeded in booking a box for the day. He invited RT to be his guest. It was a wonderful day. The boxes at Lord's are fully supplied with polite servants, flowing alcohol and lavish food. There was a constant stream of visitors. The Prime Minister was sitting in the next box. And England was beating the West Indies.

RT was very drunk by the end of the day. As we drove back to his mother's flat he started to become first maudlin and then aggressive. That evening he deliberately started an irrational argument with his mother and I had great difficulty in getting him to calm down.

The Sunday evening was even worse. The weather was very hot and he had again been entertained far too generously by JK. He was determined to have a fight with his mother. Many unfortunate things were said on both sides. Neighbours, hearing the noise, tried to intervene. RT's mother dialled 999 and then changed her mind. Eventually I got him into bed where he talked on and on for hours. He wanted to go home immediately but I persuaded him to wait until the morning.

We set off very early, listening to the last of the cricket on the car radio. He and his mother had not spoken to each other at all, but he did kiss her goodbye.

As we left London behind, so his mood lifted and he started to relax. At lunchtime he insisted on stopping at an Indian restaurant where he ordered a massive meal which he ate with great pleasure. I had never seen him eat so much.

He ate well again that evening, drank very little and talked sensibly far into the night. We discussed life, death and dying. We talked about the Ph.D.. We talked about his family. We talked, for the first time, about my future.

That ferocious argument with his mother seemed to have released a barrier within him. He was relaxed, stronger, brighter and much more open to real debate rather than the interminable monologues that had been his recent form of conversation.

The improvement did not last for long. As usual, the thought of the next hospital appointment brought on anxiety, depression and an aggravation of all the current symptoms. He was now feeling a sensation of blockage in his oesophagus whenever he tried to eat. Food would be regurgitated before it ever reached the stomach. The hiccups were becoming increasingly violent and exhausting while the 'rats' continued to gnaw at his guts every night. His bowels were opening a dozen or more times a day. He started taking morphine again.

The meeting with his doctor was routine. No blood tests were taken, no changes in medication. It was agreed that it would be sensible to take an X-ray of his stomach in case the blockage was physical but, apart from that, it was just carry on as before.

The summer continued to get hotter and hotter. RT felt drained by the heat. The hospital had lent us an electric fan that we now kept going all night so that he could be cool enough to sleep. The depression was taking hold again.

I discovered that the Lord's Taverners were holding a charity cricket match at a minor public school nearby, packed a picnic and hoped that the event might cheer him up. His Disabled Parking sticker allowed us to drive almost onto the pitch itself and we established ourselves near the pavilion in the shade of a majestic tree.

The cricket was gentle and RT was enjoying the day despite feeling very weak. But one event really captured his imagination. A bus full of children suffering from various sorts of disability had parked not far away. One small child, strapped into a wheelchair, appeared to be both mentally and physically handicapped. He had little control of his limbs and did not seem to be aware of his surroundings. One of the television stars in the Lord's Taverners team went straight to this child. There was no one else watching - no cameras, no fans to be impressed. This famous presenter took the child's hands and kissed them gently. He stroked the tense, knotted limbs, talking quietly all the time. The child slowly responded, became calmer and a little more aware. It was a very moving scene, a private scene of genuine love and generosity of spirit. It moved RT to tears.

The next day the post arrived at 11.30am - the usual time for deliveries in this rural neighbourhood - with a letter from the hospital asking RT to come for an X-ray that very day at 2.30pm and not to eat anything for eight hours before. The letter had been posted Second Class on the Friday for a Monday appointment.

Of course RT had already eaten breakfast but I rang the hospital, explained the situation and, as there were no more available appointments for at least a month, we decided to go ahead anyway. RT really coped very well with the stress of a hurried bath, no lunch or coffee, and a fifty mile dash to the hospital.

The X-ray showed no sign of a physical blockage. There was nothing that could respond to a practical remedy. We had to conclude that, once again, it was the depression that was causing the symptoms.

Everything carried on as before. There were good days and not so good days. The weather was too hot but mostly dry. When it rained we were flooded but it seemed impossible to speed up the bureaucracy of local government. We could not have a new bath and the special disability fittings until the work on the kitchen was done and no one could give any sort of estimate on how long that would take.

There was still no news about money for the car from the charities. Their various committees didn't meet in the height of summer. RT was starting to use morphine every evening - not the MST, the slow release tablets that made him hallucinate, but a simple, low dose pill that should stop the pain for up to four hours. He seemed to me to be taking it for the emotional lift it sometimes gave rather than for pain.

We were still going to The Convent once a week for lunch, friendship and alternative therapies. While RT had massage, I would have reflexology and vice versa. This started to infuriate him. He could not understand why I should need therapy too. He was the one who was ill. It was his disease - he was the one who was suffering, not me.

Of course I was hurt by his attitude. I knew that I needed all the help I could get. But I can, I think, understand why he needed to feel this way.

He was losing control of his life. I was his only point of stability. If I needed therapy then that must mean that I too was suffering and might crack up, leaving him to cope alone. This thought was intolerable. He had to believe that I was strong and invulnerable. He could not allow himself to consider that I might possibly need any sort of help at all. He could accept the idea of me having free therapy as a perk - just for the fun of it - as long as he made sure that I knew he thought I was jumping on his bandwagon and cheating the system.

––––––––––

We hoped that, once we had a reliable car, we could go away on a series of mini-holidays - just one or two nights in Bed & Breakfast hotels. Travelling seemed to be good for RT's depression and it would give him a chance to show me some of the places he had discovered as a roving journalist.

The weather was so good that it seemed a pity to wait for the new car. We decided to set off in our old jalopy with no clear plan in mind. After a meandering drive down the coast we found ourselves on the quayside of an old fishing port. A pub on the waterfront was offering B&B and we booked in.

Our room, the Captain's Cabin, was attractive and comfortable if rather small. The window looked out onto the water just a few yards away. We were feeling tired but happy.

I decided to take a shower but had great difficulty in getting it to work. At last some water did gush forth and, at exactly the same moment, a pile of crockery leapt off the shelf at the other end of the room to smash on the floor. We never did discover how to get hot water from the shower. Neither could we determine any reason for the suicidal crockery - but the incident made us both laugh, which was a rare occurrence these days.

There was an Indian restaurant nearby and RT was eager to see if he could enjoy a large curry again. The food was good but he felt claustrophobic, breathless and stressed. He kept getting up to go outside for some fresh air, leaving me to explain to the confused waiters that there was nothing to worry about - but they could see that he was very ill.

We returned to our room, ready for sleep. It was a Friday night. The weather was still so hot that we had to open the window wide. Of course, everyone in the crowded pub just below spilled out onto the street. They were not particularly rowdy but we could hear every word of the animated conversations that continued until past midnight. Then peace - until 6.30am when the street-cleaning machine rattled and squeaked its way towards us. Below our window it made a noisy three-point-turn before rattling itself away. Then the milk floats and the delivery lorries - each one having a different, piercing warning sound as it reversed and turned.

We gave in, got up early and went for a walk around the harbour. One such night was enough. After our full cooked breakfast, we decided to head for home.

On the way RT suddenly took us on a detour down a tiny lane. We parked on the rough grass of a deserted carpark and walked, following a clear path through dense woodland. Eventually we climbed over an old stone stile to find a small, muddy pool fed by a bubbling spring - a famous Holy Well. It was almost hidden in a thicket, but many rags and ribbons, most of them red, were tied to the branches of the trees and bushes.

Following the path, we came to the ruins of a tiny chapel. An altar stone stretched across the end wall. In one corner a stream flowed through an ancient font. There were more red ribbons and rags everywhere, attached to every available branch. There was a sense of mystery and power.

RT loved this peaceful, holy place. He had visited it many times in earlier years but I had never been here before. Now I knew that this was a place to which I would return - but that, next time, I would be alone.

When we got home RT insisted on having a barbecue. As we waited and waited for it to heat up enough to cook on, he tackled the brandy bottle, angry with his failure as a barbecue chef. A little later I found him curled up, fast asleep on the bathroom floor.

I heard some astonishing news. My sister was a very close friend of a local gay couple, N and L, who were both HIV+. L died of AIDS and N had become ill soon after with hepatitis and cancer. He was told that he had very few months left to live as he had only 10% liver function and there was nothing the doctors could do. He sought help from alternative therapists and healers.

Now he had 90% liver function, no cancer, was feeling very fit and the blood tests were showing no trace of HIV. Of course I rushed to tell RT. He responded with silence. Later he said, "I don't want to get better."

He had been ill for so long that it had become his way of life. He was afraid that if he got better he would lose his special Disabled Parking privileges. He might lose his Disability Benefits and have to sign on again at the Job Centre. He would have to get back to work on the Ph.D. It was all more than he could handle.

He wanted to feel better but could not, in his present state of continual exhaustion, begin to think about accepting the responsibilities of normal living. He picked up a book on spiritual healing that I had been reading, opened it at random, read a few sentences and threw it away, exclaiming, "Rubbish!"

He was worried about his reaction to N's recovery and we were able to discuss it at length. He asked other people about spiritual healing and agreed that, if we could find a good local healer, he would at least give it a try.

He was still seeking a spiritual adviser. He was becoming very worried about death, discussing it frequently but unable to share my beliefs. None of our local clergy seemed to be able to offer the intellectual and philosophical dialogue that he was seeking.

I spoke to a friend of mine, PS, an actress who had become one of the first women priests. She thought that her old tutor, now retired, might be just the right person but she wanted to meet RT first, just to be sure. He really didn't want to go. The thought of travelling some thirty miles to meet a woman priest did not appeal at all. But she was my friend and, as long as we paused at various pubs on the way, he would make the effort for my sake. I don't know what he was expecting but PS was not the sort of vicar he had imagined.

She is still a working actress, good looking and well groomed. She was wearing her dog-collar with a black top, high heels and a pencil slim skirt with a long slit. RT really did not know how to handle this situation, sitting in stunned silence for quite a while before PS succeeded in getting him to relax. But they did, eventually, achieve some sort of rapport and PS arranged a meeting between us and her ex-tutor, JE. He lived over 150 miles away but generously offered to come to us so that RT would not have to suffer the long journey.

What RT and JE discussed I do not know. PS and I went out for a long walk so that they could talk in private. Certainly RT seemed a little calmer after that day. JE kept in touch, though they did not meet again. He wrote long letters and sent some books. It was a relationship that meant much to RT even though he was not strong enough to write letters himself.

But he was still strong enough for the occasional outing. We went to the local airshow. We didn't go in - it would have been far too crowded and pretty expensive - but parked on the grass verge outside, level with the end of the runway. The commentary was broadcast on FM and I was able to find it on the car radio. So we sat in comfort as the Red Arrows roared over our heads.

A few days later we went to a Classic Car Show where RT was able, with the help of a stout shooting stick for frequent rests, to explain to me the finer points of all the vehicles.

At home he had suddenly discovered that he enjoyed watching old Marx Brothers films. I had many of them on video but he had never shown any interest. Now he wanted to see them every night - especially Harpo. He felt a strong kinship with that mischievous imp.

Some friends of mine, puppeteers, turned up unexpectedly. With difficulty I persuaded RT to join us in the garden for tea. As always, he made a great effort and switched on the charm. My friends were immediately captivated by his warmth and humour. They brought out some of their large puppets to meet him. A mature but still glamorous female puppet tried to seduce him, much to his embarrassment. An elderly male puppet wanted to discuss gardening and the dog puppet just wanted to play. RT was really out of his depth. He had never met puppets before and did not know how to behave. Should he treat them like people or ignore them and just talk to the operators? It was a lovely afternoon, full of love and laughter.

An appointment had been arranged at the local cottage hospital for RT to meet the Chest Specialist. RT was still terrified of being admitted to the main hospital in the city. The building is vast, modern and uncomfortable. He would no longer be the responsibility of his usual doctor but would be in the hands of strangers.

He did not know what sort of treatment to expect. Would they be able to make him better? Would he suffer much pain? Would there be any prejudice about his diagnosis? Would I be allowed to stay with him? Would he get out alive? It seemed sensible for him to meet this new consultant from the hospital, who would be in charge of his case, so that some of these fears might be dispelled.

It was a mistake. The whole visit was a disaster. The day was excessively hot and RT did not feel at his best. As we sat in the waiting area the Skin Specialist, whom we had not seen since that terrible day of diagnosis in October, rushed through. He looked harassed and ill, as though he might be on the verge of a breakdown. RT just froze, then walked outside for a smoke. He begged me to get him some water as he was feeling dehydrated and sick. The nurse was most reluctant to help but did eventually find a paper cup for me.

At last the consultant could see us. The nurse came to the front door to call RT in and yelled at him not to throw his cigarette away just there as it was too close to the oxygen tank. He couldn't understand what she was saying.

We were shown into the consulting room. This consultant was as cold and unwelcoming as the Skin Specialist had been. He seemed to have no idea why we were there. He had no awareness that patients might be frightened. He asked a few irrelevant questions and then said bluntly, "Well, when the time comes, do you want to go on a ventilator or not?"

RT did not understand the question. What was a ventilator? I explained that the doctor was asking if he should fight for RT's life to the bitter end or whether he would prefer to be allowed to die without too much medical intervention. RT was shocked. It had never occurred to him that they might just let him die. He insisted that he would want the ventilator and we left in angry silence.

RT was upset. He was angry, depressed and very frightened. Every night he drank too much and ate too little. Every day he raged and ranted on for hours. He hated this new consultant.

One night I was woken by a loud noise and yelling. I found RT, stark naked and very drunk, upside down on the stairs. He had tried to go down in the dark in search of more brandy and suddenly found himself flying. He had bruised his foot and his spine but seemed otherwise unhurt. I decided there was no point in calling an ambulance and tried to get him up. I was not strong enough to lift him. He was too drunk to help himself. Eventually I managed to roll him down the rest of the stairs to sit him on the bottom step.

He did cut back on the brandy after that but something had happened to his spirit. He remained restless, tense and quarrelsome. He was talking in his sleep again. The thought of food was repulsive, though he did manage to force himself to eat at times. He needed help.

He talked to his doctor who told him that he had already lived six months longer than expected. RT did not find any encouragement in that.

We both talked to the clinic's Stress Management Counsellor who was certainly more constructive in the help she offered. RT agreed to regular counselling which I hoped might ease some of his mental torment. We also learnt that an abbey, not too far away, had a guesthouse where we would be welcome to stay for a few days.

This really did appeal to RT He pictured himself having long soul-searching discussions with elderly monks. I made enquiries and booked us in for a four-day visit at the end of September. At least RT now had something to look forward to and we should have our new car by then.

I had heard from the charity that the money was on its way, though I still did not know how much. And we were now getting some help with the domestic bills and a small grant of £10 a week. This generosity relieved me of the day-to-day financial panic that RT could not recognise. He needed his brandy, cigarettes and cannabis. He was not prepared to consider any sort of economy in that area, but we were living on Income Support and all our savings were gone. Without that charity I would not have been able cope. I needed all my strength just to be able to remain calm and patient.

RT wanted to go to London. There was a cricket match at Lord's that he did not want to miss. His friend, JK, would be there and had promised that the wine would be flowing freely.

But this time RT didn't make it. He was too tired.

CHAPTER 5

Autumn 1995

I had been given the address of a spiritual healer, MC, who lived just a few miles away. She was not in the phone book and RT was still reluctant to discuss healing so I let the matter drop. Then, one Sunday when RT was even weaker than usual, I felt a sudden need to find her. With RT's permission, I wrote a brief note asking her to ring me and drove to the nearby village to see if I could find her house. I had to deliver the letter by hand as I couldn't bear to wait for the post.

Like most such villages, there were no street names or house numbers and I had to ask for directions before I could locate her cottage. I was told that the young man across the way, who was unloading a car, would be able to tell me where to find MC. Indeed he could as they had just that minute returned from holiday together and she was inside, unpacking. She invited me in.

MC was not on the phone because she had only recently moved into the area. She had moved her possessions here and then immediately gone away for a month. This was the very first moment that I could have contacted her and here I was, on the doorstep.

She was not what I had expected. I had assumed that all healers were middle-aged or elderly and usually rather fat. MC was very young and pretty with long, ash-blond hair. She was extremely thin. In fact she looked just the sort of woman who in earlier ages would have been burnt as a witch.

I did not tell her what was wrong with RT, only that he was very seriously ill, and made an appointment for the following day. She would make no charge for healing, though donations were always acceptable.

Though very sceptical, RT made no objection to this visit. I think he was starting to feel desperate. He was getting weaker all the time and he had, at last, realised that his doctor was not going to be able to provide him with the magic pill that would make him feel well again. Perhaps this healer could work a small miracle for him. They disappeared into her tiny healing room for an hour.

He seemed to enjoy the session and we returned several times over the next few weeks. RT said that she was able to get him to relax as soon as he sat down. That was a big achievement. The only other improvement was that his right foot, the one that had been smashed to pieces in the car crash, suddenly became warm, flexible and sensitive for the first time in 25 years.

RT allowed MC to tell me what she had found. The first thing she said was that he was exactly where he wanted to be. He had chosen to be ill and did not, at that time, want to get better, though he did say that he wanted to stay alive to keep me company. She was able to soothe his mind so that he could relax but his spirit would not allow her to heal the increasing weakness in his legs. His heart she could not approach as it was firmly locked in an iron cage.

I asked her if she knew what was wrong with him. She was confused. He had said it was leukaemia and, young as she was, she doubted her own judgement. She showed me her notes from their first session. The first line mentioned Immune Deficiency. Her instincts had given her the correct diagnosis right at the start.

RT became more reluctant to see MC when he found that he felt dizzy each time he entered the healing room and that during every session, while his eyes were closed, he would feel someone touch his arm even though MC was sitting on the other side of the room.

All his usual symptoms continued unchanged. The stomach cramps were becoming more insistent. There were alternating attacks of diarrhoea and constipation. Walking was now so exhausting that we rarely went out. His emotions were very volatile - one minute we would be arguing violently, then making up with a cuddle and immediately arguing again. He started having nightmares and panic attacks, often shouting in his sleep.

We had been given several Relaxation Tapes that he refused to listen to more than once. He said that he could not stand having someone tell him what to do and, to be fair, on most of the tapes the words and ideas were fine but the voices had irritating faults that grated on his raw nerves.

All books on healing and relaxation were tossed aside with contempt. I believed what MC had told me - he really did not want to get better unless someone could wave a magic wand and provide that instant miracle.

Red Claws suggested that a wheelchair might give him more mobility. He eagerly agreed and was excited when the first chair arrived the next day. It did not fit him well and had small wheels so that he could not steer it himself, but it allowed us to go out for our first walk for ages. We had fun that day as we learnt how to manoeuvre our way across roads, along bumpy paths and through groups of unobservant pedestrians.

Despite his drastic weight loss, RT was still very heavy for me to handle. In one place the road sloped down to a drain and it acted on us like a whirlpool. Gravity ensured that the chair was inevitably drawn down to that drain and I was simply not strong enough to do anything about it. Laughing, RT had to get out of the chair so that we could move on.

Later that night RT became emotional and frightened. He had wanted the wheelchair but it was a clear indication that his condition was deteriorating. Now that he had the chair he realised that he might never walk anywhere again.

Four charities had all given us either money or a letter promising to send a cheque direct to the garage once we had chosen our car. We knew exactly what we were looking for but, now that we were free to buy it, we couldn't find one anywhere.

I used the Yellow Pages to ring all the garages within 75 miles but still could not find what we wanted. Eventually one garage rang back to say that a car had just come in that was exactly what we were looking for. As soon as RT was up and dressed we drove the 35 miles and found the car. It was just right - but it had been sold five minutes before we arrived.

Disconsolately we looked at the other cars on the forecourt. I was prepared to go home again but RT decided he wanted to test drive a car that I had seen before but rejected because it was bright red, the one colour that RT had sworn he would never drive.

Apart from the colour, it was perfect. It had a very low mileage, impeccable pedigree, and we fell in love. We had found our car. It would take ten days for the finance to be finalised but we would be able to take delivery just before setting off to the Abbey for our four-day retreat.

RT's depression lifted, his appetite improved - life seemed worth living again. We took my mother's dog, Jenny, with us to the pub and RT walked with her along more than half a mile of country paths before collapsing exhausted in a tiny chapel just beyond the pub garden.

He often visited this chapel. It was built into the garden wall of a vicarage that had once been part of a convent. It was always deserted and RT loved to sit there quietly, sometimes lighting a candle, enjoying the ancient solidity of the stonework and the calming atmosphere of spiritual peace.

RT seemed calmer now and just a little stronger. I had to go up to London yet again and he decided that, this time, he would prefer to stay at The Convent rather than mope at home alone. I was a little worried about how he would cope, but it was only for one night and I knew that they would look after him for me.

There were several black women amongst the guests. Apparently RT, after his usual session with the brandy bottle, engaged them all in conversation. He started calling them, "My little coons," and referring to himself as "whitey trash" - the staff listened in awe, wondering what would happen but RT's charm was irresistible.

The women loved him. They talked to him for hours and all ended up in his room, making sure that he was comfortable. Only RT could have got away with it.

———————

Proudly we took possession of our bright red car. RT insisted on giving it an unnecessary extra coat of polish before we set off for the Abbey. Then he drove.

We arrived at the Abbey Guesthouse at the appointed time only to find the door locked. No one answered the bell but, eventually, another guest arrived with information. The Guestmaster had been called away and would return in about an hour. We were shown into a common-room and offered coffee before being left, tired and very tense, to fend for ourselves.

The Guestmaster, when he arrived, proved to be a friendly young monk who was also looking after a large wedding reception elsewhere in the extensive grounds. He showed us to our room before rushing away to his religious duties. We would see him again at dinner.

Our room was remarkably beautiful. The whole building, an ancient gatehouse, had only recently been restored. The craftsmanship involved was obvious. Everything was simple, solid, well designed and expertly finished.

We had been given a large room at the far end of the top floor where we would not be disturbed by other guests. Fortunately there was a lift - I had already explained by letter that RT was very ill. There were two bathrooms immediately adjacent, one of them fully equipped for disabled use.

Our only disappointment was the food. Dinner was a communal occasion with all the guests sitting at one large table presided over by the Guestmaster. There were several dishes of cold leftovers from the wedding feast - sandwiches, sausages, pasties and cakes. Not the sort of meal to tempt RT's fragile digestion. He could not face eating, nor did he feel strong enough to talk to a dozen hungry strangers, so he went to bed.

The next day was Sunday and, with RT in his wheelchair, we attended High Mass in the Abbey. As lapsed Catholics we were there for nostalgic reasons and to hear the choir, but the event was, of course, spiritually moving.

We then spent a cold and wet hour looking at steam trains and classic cars at a local show before retreating to a pub. RT was not well. He could neither drink his beer nor eat any food at all. We went back to the Abbey Guesthouse so that he could sleep for a while.

That evening RT again could eat nothing. But even I found it difficult to face those cold wedding leftovers again. I was longing for a decent hot meal. Unfortunately there were no self-catering facilities available and RT was not strong enough for us to go out. But he did manage to attend the evening service, Compline.

It was an extraordinarily moving experience. The Abbey was in darkness. The black-robed monks entered and sang the first part of the service in the dark. Then, gradually, candles were lit and the altar became visible. The ceremony ended with all the monks and congregation gathered together in the tiny Lady Chapel for the final chants. It was such a theatrical event that we went again every night of our stay. It never failed to stir the emotions.

That night RT started vomiting. He felt very poorly indeed in the morning. The Guestmaster asked me how RT was and I took the opportunity to tell him of the diagnosis and of RT's need for a spiritual adviser. We arranged that they should meet privately the following day.

Despite his exhaustion and nausea, RT came out with me for a wheelchair walk around the grounds. It was a beautiful day but he could find little enthusiasm. His muscles were so weak that he was finding it difficult to keep his eyelids raised - not because he was sleepy, the muscles simply would not work.

After Compline RT vomited again as I wheeled him back to the guesthouse. He couldn't swallow his pills. Then diarrhoea struck. It was a bad night. He had a long meeting with the Guestmaster the following day and seemed much calmer afterwards.

There were fewer guests now and RT felt able to sit with us in the Common Room. One lady, C, managed to get him talking and his spirits immediately rose. He was always at his best with an appreciative audience. We both had a better night.

When the time came to leave next morning, C appeared with a farewell gift of a beautifully decorated card - an illuminated quote from Cardinal Newman. She hugged and kissed RT warmly. He was captivated by her. He was convinced that she was an angel sent by 'The Management' to give him comfort and the courage to fight on.

We returned home via the clinic where we had our usual monthly appointment to see his doctor. This time some drastic changes were made to RT's pill regime but I could not concentrate enough to understand why. The biggest change was the removal of that experimental and highly toxic drug against CMV. I was glad he was to come off it but wondered why - was he now clear of CMV? Was the drug damaging his blood?

The doctor reminded us how ill RT had been when he had first entered the clinic, saying, "I thought, when I saw those terrible sores, I know what this is - but what am I expected to do about it?" He really had believed that RT would die very quickly.

That evening, as I was just starting to prepare a meal, I suddenly had to rush to the bathroom. I was vomiting violently and simultaneously attacked by diarrhoea. I was sweating, shaking and in a state of panic.

As soon as I could I yelled for RT to help me. He took one look and fetched my mother. When I was able to move away from the bathroom for a moment they took me next door where my mother could look after both of us. I just about managed to explain RT's pill regime to her before I collapsed completely. I spent all of that night in her bathroom and then slept for two days.

When I woke the next-day-but-two, my mother was vomiting and had diarrhoea - not quite as violently as I had, but she was obviously feeling awful. I asked RT to go to The Convent for two nights to give us a chance to recover; found the strength to pack his pills and a few clothes; gave him the car keys and kissed him goodbye before collapsing back into bed. When he returned we were both feeling better and just starting to be able to eat again.

RT was looking really happy when he came home. It had been very good for his self-esteem that, in a crisis, he was able to take the car and look after himself. He said that he had thoroughly enjoyed the drive home. The sun was shining; his spirits were high and life seemed worth living.

His new wheelchair arrived - in shiny red paint and grey upholstery, exactly the same colours as the car. It was made-to-measure and had large wheels so that he could propel himself. And a Parker-Knoll Recliner chair was delivered, courtesy of the Macmillan Services, so that he could sit in comfort.

We drove to a Superstore to buy some good polishes and cleaners for the car and RT seized the opportunity to practice manoeuvring himself in his wheelchair. He soon got bored inside the shop. I saw him head for the exit where a kindly customer held the door open for him. Just beyond the door was a ramp. RT had not yet mastered the art of braking and the wheelchair sped down the ramp and across the path of an oncoming car. Fortunately they did not collide and the wheelchair came to rest against some bushes.

As the long dry summer came to an end, so the floods started again. I had managed to get the council to push a rod through the drain to clear it and they insisted that there was no blockage - but still the water poured through the house.

Various builders had come to assess the problems and to submit estimates. The entire kitchen floor would have to come up so that a new drain could be laid. At least the new floor would be level and I would now have the chance to install some fitted units. The new bath and disabled fixtures would be put in at the same time as the kitchen work - but I still had no idea when that might be. I was getting angry at the delays. I tried arguing, threatening and even crying - but bureaucracy cannot be hurried.

RT could no longer bathe alone. He was not strong enough to get himself out of our tiny but deep bath without falling over. He was so tall, bony and uncoordinated that I had great difficulty in helping him and he did fall over several times despite my best efforts.

He was also too weak to dress himself. He could do it if he had to, but it took ages and exhausted him. We rarely went swimming now. He seemed a little weaker each day. The nausea was constant. He would try to vomit but his stomach was empty. There were frequent, violent cramping pains in his guts.

He was feverish all night and feeling so ill that he wanted to go into hospital. I called out the GP - the urine infection was back. He responded quickly to the antibiotic and 24 hours later his bladder was working well, the chest pains and nausea had eased and he was able to eat again. But he had been very frightened. He became panicky, angry and anxious - then delirious and manic, unable to sleep until 4.30am. I later found that he had drunk a whole bottle of brandy.

When he woke he felt very ill indeed but the GP was, understandably, not sympathetic. The brandy would destroy the effect of the antibiotic and damage RT's immune system even further. RT did cut down on the alcohol and slowly improved. He was now taking a low dose of Valium to try to calm his anxiety and that did seem to help.

Boredom was setting in. The same old symptoms every day. The weather getting too cold for gardening. His legs too weak for walking more than a few yards. Stairs were becoming a serious problem. He was so bored that he started coming out shopping with me, waiting in the car while I went into the shops - at least it was a change of scene. Occasionally he would feel fit enough for an outing to local beauty spots.

We had been invited to a wedding reception. RT insisted that we would go despite his increasing weakness. He took great pains to dress well for the occasion and to ensure that his shiny red wheelchair was looking clean and polished.

We made a dramatic entrance, pushing the chair through the crowds of guests until we reached the happy couple. Then RT made a supreme effort and stood up to kiss the bride. For a whole hour he managed to be his old, charming and entertaining self before asking to be taken home to bed.

He was drinking less and making a serious effort to be pleasant company. We would sit and talk for hours. Slowly he was coming to understand that his depression was causing at least some of his symptoms and he agreed to see a Counsellor and a Psychologist to see if they could help in any way.

Predictably RT was extremely tense and anxious when we went to see the Psychologist. Special arrangements had been made for us to meet him at the clinic, which was officially closed that day. RT was moving very slowly and we were late, so I rushed on ahead to get the locked main-door open and let RT in through the nearer side entrance. I was greeted by the Psychologist who looked at me with some confusion as though I had no right to be there. I explained that RT was having difficulty walking from the car and pushed past him to open the side door.

RT looked very old and grey as he came in, leaning heavily on his stick. The Psychologist greeted him without warmth and my heart sank as they disappeared into the consulting room. Half-an-hour later the Psychologist grimly invited me to join them. I wondered what had gone wrong but it was just that RT, knowing his memory was poor, had asked for me to be present.

The Psychologist explained that he considered RT to be suffering from Post Traumatic Shock Syndrome. The root cause was the brutal way that the original diagnosis had been pronounced and the condition had been made worse by the clumsy approach of the Chest Specialist. He wanted to try a new treatment, Eye Movement Desensitisation, that was working well with victims of rape. But for them, their trauma was in the past whereas RT's suffering was ongoing. Every day he woke to the horror of remembering that he had the 'Gay Plague'. It was not at all certain that this new therapy could help him.

RT was not convinced. He did not think his trauma was anything like that suffered by a rape victim. The treatment would require two hours of concentration on the scenes he most wanted to forget and he was sure he did not have the strength for such a long session. He was already exhausted after just thirty minutes of talking about his feelings. He agreed to make an appointment but I knew he did not really intend to keep it.

The Counsellor was more successful. For a start, she was a pretty woman and that helped enormously. She was warm, welcoming, careful and caring. RT fell in love with her on the spot. For her he would talk about his feelings. For her he would try the breathing and relaxation exercises - at last I could find a reason to hope again.

But not for long. The urine infection returned, this time with some pain around the kidneys. He was vomiting frequently and his mouth was unpleasantly dry. He seemed to respond to the antibiotic and was feeling a little better despite some heavy nose-bleeds.

I prepared one of his favourite meals of chicken, rice and peas. For the first time in weeks he was able to eat with enjoyment - then, without warning, he simply vomited all over his plate.

His doctor was shocked at the sudden deterioration in RT's condition and called in the Community Care Nurse. For the third time in a year I was quietly told that RT had entered the terminal stages of the disease and that nothing could be done but to make him comfortable. The doctor said, "The best thing would be if he got pneumonia."

But RT had not given up yet. He insisted on having his full hour of Reflexology before going home and then, after a siesta and no alcohol, succeeded in eating a full meal. But the night was very disturbed. He could not stop talking. He said it was just like being given the diagnosis all over again. Suddenly he realised that death might be very near and that his doctor was not going to help him.

He made me promise that, no matter what happened, I would never give up hope, never allow them to 'pull the plug', even if he begged for release. He knew that at times he longed to die. But he also knew that he was quite likely to change his mind a few hours later.

Early next morning the clinic rang to say that RT's blood test had shown that he was seriously anaemic, another predictable side effect of those highly toxic, experimental pills he had been taking for CMV. A blood transfusion had been arranged and I was to take him at once to the hospital.

It was an awful journey. He was so grey and weak. He sat there limply, groaning and wheezing all the time with his mouth gaping open. I thought he was dying. But when we reached the hospital he tried to insist on walking in rather than use the wheelchair - he didn't want to make a fuss.

Fortunately I was able to make him change his mind. The hospital is vast, resembling an airport in its soulless luxury, and the walk from the door to the lift would have defeated him.

We were put into a small side-ward by ourselves and RT got into bed. Then came the various doctors, nurses and other staff, each with a clip-board and a mass of questions. Apparently, despite all the blood tests that had been done over the past two years, no one had any record of RT's blood group. A sample was taken and the blood for transfusion would arrive tomorrow, but, because the doctor would not be on duty then, the needle was inserted straight away and taped into place so that any nurse could just plug in the drip as soon as the blood arrived.

The hospital food was uneatable. Even my healthy appetite rebelled at such tasteless mush. The window would only open for three inches and looked onto a blank flat roof with no greenery to be seen. Smoking was strictly forbidden except in the smoking room. The needle in RT's arm was uncomfortable. The bell to summon a nurse was fixed just outside our door and rang loudly every time a patient pressed his bellpush for attention.

With RT seated in his wheelchair, we decided to search for the smoking room. This proved to be a major expedition. First we had to get back to the centre of the building to find the lifts, then down three floors. After asking for directions, we headed off down a blank corridor. It went on and on, with no doors, posters, heating or signs. At the end we found a tiny, cold cell packed with hard benches - the smokers' punishment block.

We complained to the Staff Nurse that RT was really not well enough to suffer that journey and discomfort every time he needed to smoke. A message had arrived from the clinic that RT was not to be prevented from drinking or smoking, so brandy was prescribed for him (but not provided on the National Health) and we were shown a small fire-exit onto a staircase where the occasional cigarette would be ignored.

I had, long ago, promised RT that I would never leave him alone in a hospital. A nurse brought me a pillow and a blanket. I slept, as best I could, in an armchair at his side.

The blood did not arrive until mid-afternoon the following day. Six units had been prescribed but the blood bank could only provide five - it would just have to be enough. Slowly the blood dripped while RT prayed that this would provide the miracle he was seeking.

We were released the next afternoon. There was no instant improvement. He was still vomiting without warning, still too weak to climb the stairs. The weather was stormy and the cottage was flooding worse than ever. I was beginning to crack under the strain.

Over the weekend RT developed a raging sore throat. The white coating of candida was clearly visible. Thick catarrh was clogging his sinuses and throat making him cough and choke, which started him vomiting again. He was not eating at all. On the Monday he was worse and the GP prescribed new medication but, by the next morning, he could no longer swallow even a few drops of water without choking and was obviously dehydrated.

The GP took one look in his mouth, now completely covered with white fungus and told us that the time had come to go back into hospital. But we had a choice. We could return to that awful monstrosity in the city or go to the hospice.

We chose the hospice.

CHAPTER 6

Winter 1995

It was a decision that I had always known would come one day - but not yet! I knew the hospice well. My father had died there in 1988. It is a wonderful place, but . . .

To be driving RT there seemed to be too final; an admission, at last, that he was not going to get better.

I knew perfectly well that some patients went back to the hospice regularly over a period of years. This was not necessarily the end. RT had candida and dehydration. They were both things that could be dealt with and he would probably improve enough to be home for Christmas and our wedding anniversary.

RT was too ill to talk much on the way. We travelled in silence, each trying to cope with our own fears.

The hospice is a modern, purpose built bungalow set on a hill, surrounded by beautiful gardens. I drove up to the main door and unloaded the wheelchair. By the time I had helped RT into the chair some members of staff had arrived to welcome us. Now RT found the strength to speak.

"Do you let people out of here again?" he whispered. No wonder he had been so silent on the journey. He had never been to a hospice before. He had heard about them. They were places where you went to die. He did not know what to expect but felt too ill to be really frightened.

The staff laughed and reassured him. Patients usually stayed for two weeks on their first visit so that their condition could be assessed and their medication adjusted. He would soon be feeling more comfortable.

We were shown into our room. We could not have asked for better accommodation in the most expensive private clinic. We had privacy, space, our own bathroom, television and attractive furnishings. One wall was entirely made of glass with a french window that opened out onto a verandah, the gardens, the fields and then, in the distance, the town.

A doctor came to see us just minutes after we arrived. She looked into RT's mouth and exclaimed, "Oh, you poor chap!"

All RT's pills were confiscated. From now on they would take complete control of his medication - starting by cutting out almost everything to see what happened. A saline drip was set up and, at last, some fluid was getting into RT's system. He started to relax but he was still coughing up this flood of thick choking mucus that seemed to be trying to drown him.

We were both exhausted. The sleepless nights, the emotional decision to come here, the sudden complete removal of all responsibility for RT's welfare - it was all too much for me. I had to sleep.

The nurses produced pillows, blankets and a put-u-up chair that opened out to form a small bed. After a very pleasant evening meal, freshly cooked on the premises, I made up the bed, opened the window, turned out the lights and we both went to sleep.

Suddenly, at about 11pm, the door banged open, the lights flashed on and four strange nurses swirled into the room, filling it completely.

"Good evening! We are the Night Girls," one of them cried. She started to check the saline drip. Another began to give RT various pills and potions. The third, stepping over my floor-level bed, rushed to the window shivering, "God, it's cold in here! Is the heating working? I must shut this window and close the curtains." The fourth, after checking the settings on the heater, was in the bathroom rummaging around to find towels and some mouthwash.

We were stunned. What was happening? The only thought that came into my head was, "It's the Ride of the Valkyrie!"

After they departed we were left in peace until the morning cup of tea at 7.30am. RT was much improved. He was still coughing and choking but urine was flowing again and he was able to drink two cups of sweet tea. He was strong enough to start complaining about the restriction of being attached to a drip and the ban on smoking in the room. He hated his mattress which vibrated and rippled every few moments to reduce the danger of pressure sores.

That afternoon, while the staff changed the mattress, we went exploring. I helped RT into his wheelchair, hung onto the drip stand and manoeuvred us out into the corridor. We were seeking the Smoking Room.

It proved to be a lovely conservatory surrounded by a floodlit water garden with waterfalls and golden carp. We could have been very happy sitting there. But other patients had the same idea. They too needed to smoke and seemed to enjoy the bustle, chatter and thick atmosphere. After a swift cigarette and a few polite words, we set off on our travels once again.

We developed a method of controlling the drip stand by tucking its base under the footrest of the wheelchair. Now RT could steer it with his feet and I could concentrate on pushing.

The walls of the corridors were covered with paintings by local artists, donated to the hospice and all of them for sale. In the main concourse there was a small coffee-bar, a children's play area and a gift stall full of cards and handmade bits and pieces. One vast wall was made of glass and looked onto a tiny courtyard full of plants and benches. A fishpond extended under the glass and into the entrance hall where the fish would gather in the hope of being fed.

Eventually we found ourselves in the small, circular chapel. The walls were almost entirely made of stained glass panels. Behind the altar was a triptych of a local view embroidered onto silk panels. It was a place of light, peace and beauty. It was here that my father's body had rested the night he died.

It was another disturbed night. This time RT had diarrhoea and was making frequent trips to the bathroom, drip stand and all. But by morning he was so much better that the drip was removed and RT could have a bath. All offers of help from the staff were rejected.

"That's what I have a wife for," he insisted. The bath was fitted with an electrically controlled seat which RT at first found amusing and then annoying. It was uncomfortable for his bony bottom and made it almost impossible for him to lie down in the water. But at least there was plenty of hot water available and the pains in his limbs did ease.

After consultation with the doctor, we were allowed to go off to The Convent for his weekly massage.

He desperately needed that sign of normality returning to his life. At The Convent he could usually manage to eat at least a little. And his masseuse, AR, was one of the loves of his life. No matter how ill he was feeling, he would be eager to see 'the lovely AR' and the aromatherapy massage always soothed his spirit.

We returned to the hospice in time for the evening meal, which RT did manage to eat. Then, even though he was exhausted, he walked alone down to the Smoking Room

The improvement continued and the weather was beautiful enough for us to enjoy a wheelchair walk in the gardens. RT was getting frustrated. We had been at the hospice for only three nights but he was sure that it had been at least a week. He wanted to go home.

We came to a compromise. After a siesta we drove out to the nearest pub for a pint. Many years ago, in happier times, this pub had been RT's local. It, and the village, were full of memories of an age when life was fun, responsibilities were someone else's problem and disease did not exist.

We returned to the Hospice in time for sherry, pills and the evening meal. RT had ordered egg and chips which he ate with considerable pleasure. Then, with the windows open wide, he smoked a cigarette. A staff nurse caught him and told him off. He made no reply and, as soon as she had left, lit up again. He never could accept being told what to do.

The next morning another staff nurse came to read the Smoking Riot Act. The only effect was to increase his depression. He begged me to take him home. Instead, I took him out for lunch.

We drove to a familiar fishing village where I could push the wheelchair around the harbour while RT talked of his old memories of boats and fishermen. The sun was shining as we sat on the quayside sharing crab claws with a passing cat and a flock of importunate seagulls.

That night the coughing and choking returned. RT's bed was a sea of paper hankies as he tried, vainly, to cope with the seemingly endless mass of glutinous mucus that blocked his nose and throat. Though he was very weak, we tried another outing the next day. But it was too cold and we soon retreated to the warmth of the Hospice. RT felt very ill and miserable. He had managed another trip to the pub but he was full of aches and pains. His head hurt and he didn't want to eat. I massaged him gently until he fell asleep.

That night we were woken suddenly about 3am. A confused patient had stumbled into our room in search of a toilet. He lurched towards the bed and fell on top of RT. I leapt up and, after pushing the emergency bell, tried to help him from the room. A nurse arrived to take control and I went to make some tea - it would take some time for us to be able to get back to sleep.

By breakfast time RT seemed much brighter. A physiotherapist came to teach him some simple exercises to ease his coughing. He was eating, managed a little exercise on a 'bicycle', walked unaided to the Smoking Room and persuaded the doctor to let him go home tomorrow for three days.

Though he woke feeling fairly good, RT was angry and exhausted by the time we left the Hospice. There had been a delay of more than two hours before his pills were packed and ready for us to take home. He had no patience left to deal with such frustrations.

But, at last, we were at home again. In our absence the new bath had been fitted. The council, recognising that we had already waited far too long, allowed the work to go ahead even though we still had not had final approval for the grant for the kitchen.

RT enjoyed relaxing in his new, full-length bath. I still had to help him out as the grab-rail he needed had not yet arrived. Then we went to the pub where we bumped into a very surprised GP. He should have realised by then that nothing would keep RT away from his early evening pint.

The next morning, despite my attempts to help, RT slipped and fell in the bath, badly bruising his coccyx and his head. He was in a great deal of pain but insisted on being driven to the nearest town to do his Christmas shopping.

I parked the car at the door of the shop he had chosen and RT went in. He was moving slowly and very unsteadily.

His illness was obvious to the shopkeeper who watched over him carefully while I browsed in another room. He somehow managed to make his way upstairs and we were able to keep an eye on him on the closed-circuit video.

A few minutes later some very worried customers came down saying they thought he might need some help - but he just shooed me away. A long time later he crept down the stairs again to collapse in a chair. He ordered me to wait in the car while he described to the shopkeeper the items he had chosen. She fetched and wrapped them and then helped him into the car.

He felt very pleased with himself and, despite some severe constipation problems, continued to feel quite good until the time came to return to the Hospice. Then the anxiety and depression hit him again.

Smoking continued to be a problem. Nothing would stop RT from smoking in our room, it helped him to bring up that sticky phlegm and breath more easily. He tried to hide it but could not disguise the smell. The nurses were angry. It was their job to enforce the rule. If the fire alarm went off the whole building would have to be evacuated. Tension was building up and RT learnt to dread the arrival of any staff member.

The Convent was closed for refurbishment and he was feeling the lack of a good massage. And, of course, he wanted to see the Lovely AR. She came to the Hospice and massaged him on the bed. That eased his stress and he felt strong enough to deal with writing some Christmas cards.

RT was definitely feeling better. He even asked for second helpings of the roast pork lunch. The doctor agreed that we could go home tomorrow morning.

On this last full day of our stay we had some special visitors. Immediately after the initial, cruel diagnosis, I had telephoned LW, a very good friend whom I knew I could trust. With her I knew I could safely share our awful news.

LW lived in the city and had never met RT. She is a local television presenter, very attractive and young enough to be our daughter. We talked frequently and, just before that Christmas of '94, she met me for coffee at a half-way point between our respective homes.

We exchanged Christmas presents. I gave her a very special piece of jewellery that I had owned and loved for many years.

RT took her to his heart that night. He was watching her evening news bulletin and noticed that she was wearing that distinctive necklace that I had given her just a few hours before. He was so pleased that she had chosen to wear my gift.

A few weeks later LW came to see us both. She knew that the 'official' diagnosis was leukaemia and that RT must never realise that she knew the truth. Of course I was just a little bit afraid that she might let something slip - but I trusted her and wanted them to meet.

They became firm friends instantly. She loved his dry humour and charming manners. He was captivated by her beauty, spontaneous affection and sweet, generous nature. When she became engaged she brought her fiancé to meet us. Now they were both coming to the Hospice.

RT was excited and tense. He insisted on going to the pub before they arrived. Once back at the Hospice he started drinking brandy just to ease his stress. By the time they arrived he was very merry.

He took them to the Smoking Room to make sure that everybody knew that this well known, beautiful young woman was his friend. Anyone who failed to recognise her was immediately introduced. He was name dropping shamelessly, and having a wonderful time.

We ate dinner in the Concourse where everyone could see us. RT was now drinking sherry and wine, but not eating at all. His behaviour was becoming outrageous as he manoeuvred his wheelchair around the table, blatantly smoking in front of the staff, ignoring their reprimands.

But he was so happy. He was back in his old familiar role of perfect host and entertaining companion with an attractive and appreciative audience.

As we said our farewells, LW told me that she wished she could tell RT that she knew he had AIDS, so that he could see it made no difference to her feelings for him. She knew it could not happen - that it would have destroyed his trust in me if he knew I had revealed his secret.

Inevitably all that alcohol upset his already damaged sense of balance. He was unable to get to the bathroom without falling over. He had diarrhoea and stomach cramps. It was a rough night for both of us.

But we were going home. He awoke looking very pale but in a bright, humorous mood. Blood and urine samples were taken for testing; fond farewells were said and we left the Hospice behind.

That afternoon was busy. The Community Care Nurse came on one of his routine visits at the same time as AC, the Occupational Therapist, arrived with her technician to assess what physical aids RT now needed if we were to cope at home.

Once again RT was in his element. He sat in his great Parker Knoll Recliner and held court while his guests drank tea and allowed him to entertain them.

AC decided that we needed handrails on the stairs - both indoors and in the garden. A floor-to-ceiling pole beside the bath would provide a suitable support for RT as he struggled to climb out of the water. A bath seat would be provided, just in case it proved useful. A special framework and raised seat would be attached to the toilet. An extra step would make the steep access to our bedroom easier to manage. A grab rail beside the bed would help him balance as he stood to use his urine bottle in the night.

The bed would be raised on three-inch wooden blocks and an electric motor would be fitted beneath the mattress so that the head end of the bed could be raised or lowered at the press of a button.

What I needed AC couldn't provide. She couldn't prevent the rainwater from flooding through the whole ground floor and she had failed to get the council to speed up its decision on the grant for repairs.

I had managed to get hold of some sandbags which, together with some plastic sheeting, had reduced the speed of flow of water under the door to a rate that gave me time to move carpets and start bailing out. But that was hardly good enough. I had too much to cope with anyway. It was nearly Christmas and the weather was going to get worse. I pointed out that if something didn't happen soon I would have to ask for us to be rehoused as a matter of urgency, on health grounds.

All these visitors had made RT very animated. He needed to talk far into the night, drank too much brandy, and neither of us got much sleep. The next morning we were flooded again. RT felt inadequate, ill and depressed. He drank lots of brandy and talked about suicide.

He had a very long talk with his doctor at the clinic next day. They discussed suicide and euthanasia. His doctor explained that none of his current pills would provide a reliable lethal dose but that, when the time came that he could no longer bear to go on, he could be put on to intravenous morphine and the dosage increased until he was comfortable. There was an implicit promise to help him die whenever he felt it necessary.

It seemed likely that RT was anaemic again. It had been more than a month since the blood transfusion. Another test was taken and we were promised that, if the level proved low, another transfusion would be arranged immediately.

The doctor also insisted most firmly that RT must go onto MST, the slow-release morphine that we had instinctively resisted for the past year. It was, we were assured, a very low dose and completely harmless. No one mentioned constipation.

The MST certainly helped him to sleep. He got up once in the night, losing his balance and knocking his overloaded bedside table to the floor. He felt sleepy, but very good, all morning finally getting up at 3.30pm. Then he felt dizzy and started vomiting. He had passed no urine since the night before.

He managed to keep a little food down and seemed stronger but he was very depressed and had violent stomach cramps that kept him awake despite the MST.

The next morning and still his bladder was not working. The Macmillan nurse, who had come round to discuss his suicidal thoughts, sent for the GP. Their joint diagnosis was that the MST had, typically, caused severe constipation and the blocked bowel was obstructing the flow of urine. If suppositories did not clear the problem by 3pm then he would have to have a catheter.

Another GP, a newcomer to the practice, arrived at 2pm. The condition had not improved and he insisted on fitting the catheter. RT protested that he still had an hour to go, but the GP was not to be dissuaded.

He was obviously just out of hospital and not yet used to home visits. He still expected to have a nurse at his elbow with everything prepared. He started to fit the catheter together only to realise that he had not unwrapped everything and had no sterilised surface on which to put things.

He asked me to help and together we got the catheter kit assembled and inserted. The bag immediately filled with a whole litre of urine and RT felt much better until he was told that the catheter would not be removed for at least five days, not until after the Christmas holiday. He was distraught.

The young GP had not brought a leg bag. The one he had fitted had a very long connecting tube and was obviously intended to go on a stand which we did not have. The GP had suggested tying it in place with a tape, but that was clearly not going to work. Also, he had given me no instructions on cleaning the bag. Was it supposed to stay in place for five days without being changed?

I rang the District Nurse and she came round at once, armed with boxes of spare bags, short tubes and properly designed leg straps. At least RT would not be confined to the house - we could get out to the pub.

The next day was our wedding anniversary. RT was still in pain, still suffering from constipation. He felt utterly miserable but forced himself to get up in the afternoon so that he could buy me a present.

I went next door to tell my mother that we were going out. I returned to find him trying to reverse the car out of the drive. He had got the angle completely wrong and was now attempting to drive forward through a rough slate wall. The stones were scratching the bumper and he was in a state of panic, unable to work out what was going wrong. With difficulty I persuaded him to let me drive. He slumped into the passenger seat in despair. He had suddenly understood that he would never drive again.

I dropped him off at the shop he had chosen and went to park the car. When I returned with the wheelchair there was no sign of him. The shop was locked despite the large sign saying 'Open'. Where was he? There was another shop he might try but it was across the road, up a steep incline, over a bridge and then down some steps. Surely he could not have walked that far.

I rushed to that shop and peered through the window. There he was, collapsed in a chair while something was being wrapped up on the counter. It did not matter to me what present he had chosen or how much it might have cost - the extraordinary effort it must have taken for him to have walked those few yards was a true measure of his love.

Despite the anger and frustration that he must have felt when he discovered the first shop was closed, he had not given up. He had struggled to reach the other shop and searched for a present he thought suitable.

He then refused to give it to me. He had become confused about dates and thought our anniversary was tomorrow, Christmas Eve. When I was allowed to open the parcel I found a beautiful, funny pair of dragon bookends. It was the last present he would ever buy me and the best he had ever chosen. I can see them as I write.

On Christmas Eve, at last, the constipation responded to treatment. At RT's insistence, I rang the GP but he was adamant that the catheter must stay in place for another three days. In desperation RT turned to the brandy. He drank far too much and became argumentative.

He started falling over. He fell going upstairs; he fell in the bathroom so that I found him stuck with his head trapped between the toilet and the wall; he fell out of bed with his head in the wastepaper bin. He could not understand what the catheter was for and kept trying to get up to go to the toilet for a pee. We got no sleep at all until 4am.

Christmas itself was very quiet. We were both exhausted and RT seemed confused. We attempted a wheelchair walk in the sunshine but the wind was bitterly cold and we gave up after a few yards.

We visited my mother and RT just sat, drinking too much and eating too little. At bed time he was wanting to talk but made little sense. He was ordering me to remove the catheter. When he finally stopped arguing and went to sleep I sat downstairs and cried. I thought about ringing the Samaritans but could not face explaining everything.

We were flooding every other day now. The carpets were permanently rolled up and the floor was covered with a thick layer of newspapers - the spare copies of those newspapers we had so lovingly written and published in what now seemed a different lifetime. There were piles of rags, old rugs and towels at strategic points in an attempt to control the flow of water and channel it away from electrical equipment and furniture.

I was frightened and lonely. Christmas seemed to go on for so long. All our usual support services had closed down for the holidays and, except for emergencies, we would see no one for two whole weeks.

RT slept most of Boxing Day. Then, when he got up for a bath, we found blood in the urine bag. Was it serious? Should I call the doctor?

Eventually I rang the Macmillan Service and spoke to the Duty Nurse. We discussed his symptoms and she decided that there was no immediate cause for worry. He had probably just been pulling at the tube and damaged the lining of the bladder. It would get better by itself. RT still seemed very confused.

The very first thing, next day, I rang the District Nurse to make sure that she remembered she was supposed to come to remove the catheter.

She knew nothing about it. In all the pressure of Christmas emergencies, the GP had forgotten to mention it to her. After various frantic phone calls and apologies she arrived at 10.30am with strict instructions that he must be peeing properly by 4.30pm or the catheter would go back.

RT tried to drink. He managed some tea and a few cold drinks, but not enough really. He tried to urinate, but nothing happened. He was desperate. At 4.15pm he told me that he had just been to the bathroom and that his bladder was now fine. I asked him if he was sure and he insisted that he had managed a really good pee. So I rang the GP and said that all was well.

We went to the pub and heard the GP speaking in the next bar. RT became very agitated and we went home. Then, in tears, he admitted that he had lied. His bladder was still blocked and he was very frightened. Would he have to go to hospital? He couldn't bear to have the catheter put in again. He found it all so uncomfortable and embarrassing. He hated watching me change the bag. We agreed to wait until the morning before taking any action.

I was worried. I knew that his kidneys could become infected if the bladder was blocked for too long. But I had promised to wait. Then, at midnight, he managed to pass a small trickle. Not enough but at least a sign that the blockage was not complete.

He was coughing all night and, once again, drowning in the copious, sticky phlegm. By morning he was peeing well but feeling sick and frail. He was too weak for me to massage his legs - all I could do was stroke them gently. He drank lots of water, coughed all day, and asked me to get the GP to come round tomorrow morning.

The GP was encouraging. He checked RT's chest and could find no sign of pneumonia. We discussed the problem of the Death Certificate and he promised to do some research. If it was permissible to avoid using the word AIDS on the certificate itself he would do so. He had not heard the results of the recent blood tests so we still did not know if RT's increasing weakness was due to anaemia. And he told RT quite firmly that if he did not start eating again he would die very soon.

That night RT suddenly developed a very high fever. I gave him some aspirin and his temperature dropped. He had no sense of balance and dropped his urine bottle. I went to the chemist next day and managed to buy a special valve for it so that, if he dropped it again, at least it would not spill.

RT tried desperately to eat but could manage no more than a few mouthfuls. Then I found that he had drunk a quarter of a pint of Cod Liver Oil. He had always enjoyed the taste and could not understand that too much was not good for his damaged digestive system. Once again he retreated into alcohol.

He fell over, tangled up in various chairs. With difficulty I got him back onto his feet. A little later he lurched into the kitchen in search of more brandy and fell over, dragging the marble bread board, sharp bread knife and a large cast-iron frying pan down with him. I was getting very angry.

He slowly dragged himself upstairs and I heard a crash. I found him lying outside the bathroom with a nasty cut close to one eye. His lip was also bleeding and so was a knee. He was, briefly, unconscious and had no recollection at all of falling.

Again, he had a sudden fever in the night. He felt sick and was still coughing.

The next day was New Year's Eve. He stayed in bed. He was coughing all the time and passing urine much too frequently. The fever returned and then a drenching sweat that left the bed completely soaked. His speech seemed to be slurred all the time and he was confused, the candida was returning, he was not eating and vomiting up whatever he drank, his weight was dropping and he was getting weaker every day, his breathing was getting shallower, his pulse was too fast. I could not let him out of my sight because he kept falling over.

It was past midnight - New Year's Day. And it was raining again.

I could no longer cope. I stood at the top of the stairs in the middle of the night. I was hugging the wall and crying . . .

"Help me! Please, somebody help me!"

CHAPTER 7

January 1996

In the morning of New Year's Day RT seemed much better but I knew that I had come to the end of my resources. I could no longer look after him at home. I rang the Macmillan Service and asked if we could go back to the Hospice. It was all arranged within minutes. RT accepted my decision without argument. I packed some essentials and we set off.

When we arrived at the Hospice we were greeted by Matron. I left her to wheel RT inside while I parked the car. I returned to find them both in deep conversation.

RT had informed Matron quite firmly that he intended to smoke in his room. He offered to push his bed over to the window so that he could keep his arm outside but nothing would stop him from smoking.

Matron asked why he could not use the smoking room as the staff were happy to push his bed there whenever he wished. He explained that the smoking room was too full of people and smoke The television was always on. The windows were never open and he was expected to make pleasant conversation.

He also explained that he never smoked a whole cigarette. He would just light up, take a few puffs and then start coughing. That was the whole point. He needed to cough to clear some of that thick phlegm that was making it so hard to breath but it was not a pleasant sound or sight. He could hardly inflict that on his fellow patients in the smoking room.

Matron accepted his arguments and left us while she consulted with the rest of the staff. A short time later she arrived with an ashtray and the smoke alarm was switched off. RT was the very first patient in the history of the Hospice to be allowed to smoke in his room.

This decision transformed RT's relationship with the staff. Now he no longer had to try to hide his cigarette. He need not fear each opening of the door, expecting a reprimand. He was able to make friends with the nurses and to welcome their attentions.

Of course there were some little accidents. He kept falling asleep with a cigarette in his hand. Mostly he burnt holes in his pyjamas or himself, but there was some damage to the blankets and the floor. A protective covering was put down in the danger zone and we all tried to watch carefully so that he did not burn himself too badly.

Soon after we had settled back into our old room the doctor arrived. She immediately diagnosed a return of the dehydration and a saline drip was set up. RT became feverish and confused. In my diary I wrote, "Thank God we are here!"

The sense of relief was enormous. I was no longer alone. Here, in this beautiful building, there were only a few patients - usually about fifteen - but I counted four doctors and some forty nurses on the various shifts, as well as all the auxiliaries and volunteers. And my welfare was part of their concern. My exhaustion was noticed and a bed was set up in the neighbouring music room so that I could have a quiet refuge of my own but I was not yet ready to leave RT's bedside for more than a few minutes.

That first night was bad. RT had diarrhoea and, much to his embarrassment, soiled his sheets and pyjamas. He was awake all night coughing, going to the bathroom and just talking endlessly.

Mostly it was nonsense but then came the insults. I had heard it all before and knew that he was simply using me as a punchbag. He was frightened and angry, losing all control of his life. Attacking me was the only thing he could do to prove that he still existed, still had some power, that he was more than just a patient, a body to be washed, dressed, fed and drugged whenever the nurses chose.

By morning it was clear that the saline drip was really helping. RT was much stronger already. He wanted a bath and the nurses offered to take him for a Jacuzzi. He agreed, not knowing what was involved.

A special chair was brought to the bedside. RT had to sit sideways on it and be strapped in. It was all far too confusing for him and he complained bitterly. He couldn't understand what was happening.

We pushed the large chair and the drip stand along the corridors to a bathroom where there stood a vast bath that looked more like a boat. It was already full of water being kept at a constant temperature. A button was pushed and the bath lowered itself.

We removed RT's clothes and strapped him into the chair again. Then the chair lifted and swung out over the bath. The button was pushed again and the bath came up around RT. The chair was removed to leave RT lying completely flat in the water.

RT loved the gentle massage provided by the strong Jacuzzi jets but he could not accept the presence of nurses in the bathroom. He argued and fought all the way. It was with considerable relief that we finally got him dried and dressed and back into bed.

A little later he insisted on being disconnected from the drip so that he could go to the pub. The doctors seemed surprised but agreed.

He enjoyed that pint and we spent a very pleasant hour sitting together, talking of nothing in particular. But that evening, after some brandy, he again became argumentative and abusive. The nurses insisted that I should leave him and sleep in the music room.

Of course I felt guilty but I knew I had to sleep. The nurses promised to keep a close watch on him and I closed my door - alone for the first time for longer than I could remember.

I slept well but woke very early and immediately went to check on RT. He was feverish. The doctor thought it might well be the urine infection returning - or a chest infection - or both - and he was put back on the antibiotic.

The fever continued all day and he became very confused. He demanded a shower. I knew he meant a bath but he insisted that he wanted a shower. He became upset when the nurses refused to take him into our own bathroom, which did not have a shower, but sat him in the wheelchair and pushed him down the corridor to the shower-room. Again he was affronted by the presence of nurses. It was his wife's job to help him. And he hated showers. He needed to soak in a hot bath - but he could not understand that he was still using the wrong word.

We had a similar confusion later in the day. He was adamant that he wanted scrambled eggs and black sauce. He was horrified when the meal arrived. He had thought he was ordering egg and chips with brown sauce. He refused to eat anything but did drink the pint of beer I had fetched from the pub.

With encouragement from the staff, I decided to sleep in the music room again and woke to find RT looking much better. The saline drip was removed, blood tests were taken, the coughing had eased and RT was able to eat with some enjoyment. He asked me to take him down to the physiotherapy room where he exercised his legs gently on the bicycle machine.

The relationship between RT and his mother had improved greatly since that blazing row in the summer. She would ring us up most evenings to ask me how he was feeling. Sometimes he would talk to her himself and, while they would never really understand each other, a deep affection was becoming apparent on both sides.

I had, of course, told her that we had returned to the Hospice. She was not well enough to visit us but RT spoke to her on the phone every day. His brother, JD, decided to take a day off work to drive to the Hospice - a round trip of 500 miles. He tried to persuade their mother to come with him but, sensibly I think, she realised that, much as she wanted to see RT, she would not be able to cope with such a long journey.

RT was very anxious about seeing his brother. There was a large age gap between them and they had never been close friends. The Community Care Nurse was due to visit us the same day and RT was terrified that he might talk to JD and accidentally let slip that RT did not have leukaemia. I promised to do my best to keep them apart.

The latest blood tests had shown that RT was anaemic again and just a few minutes before JD was due to arrive a blood transfusion was set up. The effect was remarkable. RT visibly improved as the blood went in. There was more colour in his face and hands. He seemed more alive.

JD arrived and all RT's anxiety evaporated. They were soon chatting happily together. Over lunch I had a chance to get to know my new brother-in-law, whom I had only met on that one brief occasion at their mother's flat.

He asked many searching questions about RT's illness. I wished I could tell him the truth. He seemed the sort of person who would understand. But I had given my word.

The Community Care Nurse arrived late enough that I was able to take him off for coffee and leave RT and JD alone to make their farewells. He had never been to this Hospice before and was delighted to have a chance to look round.

He assured me that we were in the right place. Despite their relative lack of experience in dealing with this disease, the doctors here would have much more skill in controlling RT's pain than anyone at the clinic.

It was a relief to talk to someone who had known RT since our first visit to the clinic, who could see the changes in him and who could, perhaps, understand some of the pressure that had driven me to ask for us to be readmitted to the Hospice. RT could not understand. He wanted to be at home and blamed me for forcing him to stay here.

He was too confused to listen to my reasons. In despair I sat beside him as he dozed and wrote in my diary. At the top of the page I put a heading - 'Why I can't cope at home' - then a list of all the problems. They filled the whole page.

First I mentioned his confusion and hallucinations. I found them very frightening. I am a logical person who finds it difficult to handle irrational arguments without resorting to anger.

Then there was his lack of control over his cigarettes. At home that would be very dangerous indeed. Our ancient cottage would be very vulnerable to fire and I could not be at his side all the time.

At home he would refuse to eat. It was so easy for him just to say, "No. I'll try to eat something later." In the Hospice food was brought at regular times and he at least tried to eat some of it.

In bed at home he became bored and depressed - the room is small and dark with no space for a television. He was too weak to use the stairs or go to the bathroom unaided. Here we had space, light and luxury. There were no stairs to negotiate. The bathroom was just two paces from the bed. The view was stunning and help was always available.

At home he would try to relieve the boredom with alcohol. He would insist on going to the pub. By the time we got home again he would be cold and exhausted - much too tired to try to eat anything. He would then demand brandy and drink himself into a rage, fall over and injure himself. Then we would argue and I would cry myself to sleep only to be woken at 3am when he fancied a cup of tea or another night sweat had drenched the bed and the linen must be changed.

And with all of this I would still have to deal with the floods.

Writing it all down did help to ease the guilt that RT had tried to make me feel. Once it was on paper I could see the impossibility of struggling on as we had over Christmas. Somehow I must try to help RT to understand that here, in the Hospice, we could have more time to be together - to enjoy each other's company.

Much of the time I sat on the end of RT's bed. There were pillows for me to lean against and I could stretch my legs out alongside RT's body to tuck my toes into his armpit. It was a comfortable, intimate, relaxed position. Sometimes we gently stroked each other's legs as we talked.

He looked at me and asked, very seriously, "What do you regret most?" I thought for a moment before replying.

"That the lovely person that you really are has not had a chance to develop," I said. RT nodded in approval. He understood what I meant.

Through this illness he had learnt to be able to show his true feelings. There were times when he could be openly loving, trusting and generous. His acceptance by the University had at last proved to him that his writings were worthwhile, that he was intelligent and could make a valuable contribution to research in his chosen field. He was no longer just a Good Time Charlie or a Deb's Delight.

But now he knew he would never write again. Frustration, fear and constant pain frequently drove him to anger. Our moments of mutual loving affection had become quite rare.

I treasured these quiet times spent, mostly in silence, sharing a hospital bed.

One morning, when I woke early in the Music Room and went to check on RT, I found him lying on his bed fully dressed. He had, apparently got up at about 5am and given himself a bath. He was confused. He was convinced that it was the evening and was angry that I had not yet taken him to the pub. He was also complaining of double vision and was having great difficulty in controlling his hands enough to light his cigarettes. He was certain that I had promised we would be going home tomorrow.

My mother rang. It was raining heavily and the water was pouring in faster than she could handle. A letter had arrived from the Council saying that the grant for the work in the kitchen had finally been approved. The builders had called to say they would start work tomorrow.

I had to go home. I tried to explain to RT but he was too confused to understand. So I explained to the staff nurse and left him in her care.

Everything had to come out of the kitchen. All the food, crockery, utensils, bottles of wine and bits of equipment had to be put into boxes and bags and piled high, above flood level, in the living room or upstairs. Room had to be found in the living room for the freezer, fridge, cooker and washing machine while leaving a clear, wide path for the builders between the front door and the kitchen. Cupboards and the sink could be stored in the garage.

How could one small kitchen contain so much stuff? Together, my mother and I did what we could. We did not have enough boxes or sufficient strength to finish the task. I would return the next morning with more boxes and we would have to hope that the builders would help.

RT was more lucid that evening and I was able to get him to understand that we no longer had a home that we could live in. We would have to stay at the Hospice until the builders had finished. He understood but was very upset. He begged me to stop sleeping in the Music Room. He hated being on his own and wanted to have me at his side in the night. Of course I agreed.

The next day he seemed brighter than usual and made no complaint when I left for home to sort things out with the builders. But he refused all offers of food until I returned soon after lunchtime. Then he did try to eat a little. He was very weak but unusually affectionate. I lay on the bed and we talked.

He was tired of being so ill. He wanted to give up and die. We did not know if he could get better. No one knew.

At the Hospice almost all the patients are suffering from cancer. The doctors can recognise each stage of the disease and predict its likely progression.

With AIDS it is different. I knew of many cases where the patient had apparently been in a worse state than RT and still made a dramatic recovery. The urine and chest infections could be brought under control. If he could start eating properly then he might be able to regain some weight and strength. If only he could find some reason for hope then he might stand a chance.

All last summer he had dreaded the coming of this winter. He knew that, with the shorter hours of daylight, his spirits would sink. He did not believe that he would see the spring. But I had promised him that I would never give up hope. I had to go on fighting for him, to trust that we did have a future together.

RT's anaemia had stabilised. His haemoglobin level was no longer falling. A new antibiotic was added to try to deal with the persistent urine infection. His chest seemed clearer and he was much less confused.

There were signs of pressure sores on his buttocks and the nurses gave him a different mattress to see if it would help. His nose suddenly started bleeding uncontrollably and he needed yet another drug to help the blood to clot. His body looked just like a skeleton covered with skin.

Our local vicar, Rev. R, came to visit. We had met him a few times in the past months. He was fairly new to the parish and a great improvement on the previous incumbent. Ordained quite late in life, we found he shared many of our interests and friends from his previous career. And he had made a special study of HIV. He assured RT that it was indeed possible to recover from such a weak state and promised to return in a few days to perform the Ceremony of Anointing that RT hoped might help to calm his spirit.

But still RT was giving up. His depression was deeper than ever. His skin looked grey. There were black circles round his eyes. The pressure sores were becoming painful. He showed no desire to eat anything at all.

In the Sunday papers I came across an article on François Mitterand and how he had planned his own death. On New Year's Eve he had eaten a special farewell meal with his family before retreating to his Paris flat where, refusing all food and medication, he meticulously finalised his affairs and planned his funeral before lying down to die a few day later.

I read the article to RT. He was clearly very moved. He had a long talk with the doctor who agreed that if he did not eat then he would, indeed, die very soon. She promised to find out if it would be possible to leave out any mention of HIV or AIDS on the Death Certificate, but was not at all hopeful.

I then rang his mother and insisted that he talk to her, to explain to her that he did not want to live. He was very angry with me but that seemed better than the apathetic depression of the past few days.

I left him to his anger and sat by myself in the Concourse. The Hospice Director, AA, came to sit beside me. The first member of staff to notice my need for company and support.

He had taken up his post only two weeks before and was still very much the new boy. We understood each other easily and I was pleased to have someone to talk to. The other staff seemed to be wary of intruding on the very strong relationship that so obviously existed between RT and me. My mother and some friends did visit us occasionally but most of the time we were on our own. AA quickly became a good friend and a reliable source of support.

RT was still angry the next morning and accused me of over-dramatising the situation - but he was much stronger and brighter. He talked sensibly about the Mitterand article and admitted that it had made him think about what he was doing.

That was really all I had wanted. If RT wanted to give up then that was his right. But it ought to be a positive decision not just negative lack of action resulting from despair.

The Anointing did help his spirits. He began to eat and drink again. The infections were retreating. His bottom was healing and the cough had eased. But, as a result of all the antibiotics killing off the good bacteria along with the bad, I knew the candida was returning. The doctor disagreed - it was just a dry mouth.

RT felt strong enough to go to pub again. He enjoyed the outing but was sick on the five-minute drive back. He was sick again as soon as I had got him back into bed. The nurse gave him an anti-nausea injection in the buttock - he complained bitterly of the pain.

I had been right about the candida returning. It was clearly visible in his mouth and had probably invaded his digestive system, causing much of the nausea and gut ache.

Now he was sleeping most of each day and night. The doctor drastically reduced the number of pills he was taking in an attempt to reduce the nausea. He was being woken for medication every few hours - even at 5am.

I was trying to get the nurses to understand that they did not need to rouse him each time with loud, cheery greetings that always left him confused and angry. Slowly they understood that I could wake him gently, with a kiss, just enough to swallow the drugs and go straight back to sleep.

Some of the staff had become his firm friends. They were beginning to understand his dry humour and black moods.

A few seemed more like enemies. I could see them watching me coldly as I made cups of tea, filled hot water bottles, or walked the corridors for a bit of exercise. Were they prejudiced against AIDS, or frightened for their own safety? Or was it his Public School accent or bad temper or the fact that he was allowed to smoke? Did they, perhaps, resent my competence at nursing my own husband?

Once I found RT absolutely furious. He had been in the bathroom, sitting on the toilet, when one of 'the enemy' had pushed open the door and stood over him, silently, hands on hips. When she did not move or speak he swore at her loudly and insisted that she leave at once. Which she did.

He was outraged. What the nurse was doing, I have no idea but RT's anger at her returned again and again. He could not stand her near him.

I had noticed two of 'the enemy' staring at me one day as I left the Staff Kitchen. I had been in there to make a cup of tea as there were no mugs in the coffee bar in the Concourse. A few minutes later the Staff Nurse came to ask me not to enter the kitchen because of insurance problems - the coffee bar was intended for use by patients and guests. Obviously my activities had been reported.

A few days later I went to the coffee bar to fill up two hot water bottles for RT. A volunteer was on duty making coffee for visitors. She glowered at me as I went to the sink. She snorted and sighed as she had to wait while the bottles filled. She pushed me out of the way as I tried to tighten the stoppers. I did not know what to do. I could not speak. It was such a small incident but the rejection was more than I could stand.

My expression must have said it all. AA was passing as I returned to our room. He immediately hugged me and asked what was wrong. I struggled to explain through my tears and he reassured me that I had more rights here than any volunteer.

I did not see that particular volunteer again. Perhaps she was moved to another area of work.

This was the point of no return. I knew that if RT did not start to improve over the next few days he would die very soon.

He was still capable of making the effort to talk pleasantly to his visitors. My actress friend, the Rev. PS, came to offer her love and support. And so did the healer, MC, and my mother. But as soon as they were gone he would sink back into ever deeper depression.

I discovered that he was no longer being given anti-depressants and queried the doctor's decision. The pills were restarted and his mood improved a little.

Constipation was a continual problem and RT was having to accept the indignity of suppositories and enemas. Then all the laxatives would cause diarrhoea and he would be unable to wake up enough to reach the bathroom in time.

The inside of his mouth turned dark brown. Black flakes of dead skin were rubbing off onto his toothbrush. The doctor took me aside and explained that this was necrosis. The skin was dying. The cells of his body were giving up. Once again I was told that he had entered the terminal stages. Should I believe her? Would he prove them all wrong yet again?

It was his birthday in five days. Would he still be alive? What sort of presents could I buy?

His mother had sent me a cheque. She wanted me to buy him some very expensive pyjamas. I found a beautiful pair in a sale. I also bought some bright red socks that he had always wanted and a lovely soft, old-fashioned night-shirt that I knew he would like.

In an art gallery I fell in love with a wooden sculpture of a cat. There was enough money left from his mother's present - so, after much thought, I bought it. I knew that, a few months ago, RT would have appreciated such a beautiful piece of woodwork. He would have polished it for hours. Now, the most that I could hope was that he would enjoy the feel of it in his hands for a few minutes. I bought it because I wanted it. I needed, at this difficult time, to have some beauty in my life.

There was some steady improvement all that week. He was able to read the papers again and find an interest in television. One of his favourite nurses gave him a full massage. He was eating just a little.

His birthday was a good day. The nurse he loved best helped him to open his cards and presents. He stroked the wooden cat and insisted on wearing the night-shirt and red socks after his bath. Red Claws came to visit and he enjoyed talking to her.

But in the afternoon, when we were alone, he started shouting at me to get into the car, miming shutting the door and driving. He seemed wide awake but was obviously hallucinating. I managed to get his attention. He could remember a feeling of panic but did not know why it had seemed so urgent that we should drive away.

The next day he was strong enough to get dressed to meet my mother. He was eager to learn how the builders were progressing and talked about returning home very soon. My hopes started to rise once more.

But late that evening he suddenly got out of bed and dashed through the door. He could not stand unaided but somehow managed to lurch out into the corridor to collide, head first, with a rough brick wall. He did not know where he was. His head was bleeding from a deep gash over one eye. A nurse came to my assistance and we got him back to bed.

He became very aggressive, refusing treatment for his wounds, rejecting medication. In his sleep he was talking loudly and gesturing all the time, though I could make little sense of what he was saying.

From 3am onwards he was getting up to go to the bathroom every few minutes. His bladder was hurting. He rejected all my attempts to help him, preferring to struggle alone, complaining when I lifted his legs back into the bed each time. He was abusive, unco-operative and talking gibberish continuously. Once again I found myself hugging a wall and crying for help.

In the morning the doctor took me away and explained that this really was the end. His brain and body were no longer working together. She gave him a sedative injection and put him onto a morphine driver, a little box that dripped minute doses of the drug straight into a vein every few seconds.

I rang my mother and asked her to notify RT's family and to come and be with me for a while.

Slowly the drugs worked and RT calmed down. He seemed to understand my explanations of what was happening. I told him that he was dying, that it would soon all be over. I said goodbye and he squeezed my hand.

That night, when we were on our own, I sat on the bed with his head cradled in my arms. Together we listened to his favourite music, *Spem in alium*, the 40 part motet by Thomas Tallis. To me it sounds like a choir of angels spinning a haunting tapestry of pure sound. RT relaxed.

I didn't sleep that night. The muscle relaxant injections only seemed to work for an hour and a half, then RT would get restless again and his bladder would hurt. The injections were very painful, and I would have to hold and comfort him. Despite the morphine every little movement hurt and he hated being turned over to relieve the pressure sores.

In the morning a catheter was fitted to ease the bladder pain and the morphine dosage was increased. He managed to suck some water from a sponge and fought against having a blanket bath. He was definitely aware of what was happening and fighting hard.

My mother, the Rev. R and Red Claws all came to be with us. A second electronic box was attached to him to provide the muscle relaxant without those agonising injections.

That evening I sat on the bed and talked. He took my hand and listened, obviously aware of me and my sorrow. I talked of my beliefs and described for him the Mind World I had created that I retreated to at night, before sleep. A world of beauty and healing where I could relax. I asked him to try to meet me there for a hug.

Exhausted, I went to bed. In my Mind World RT was already there. We held each other close and I fell asleep. I woke at 5am. RT's breathing was fast and shallow. I took his hand and he said, "Hallo." A little later he whispered my name twice.

He listened to me talking but seemed frightened. He tried to cough but wasn't strong enough. His breathing was rough and noisy, which seemed to worry him. The nurses insisted on giving him a blanket bath. He cried out with pain at every movement. Then they cleaned his mouth and turned him slightly onto one side. His breathing seemed easier now.

His eyes were sticky so I bathed them explaining that it would make it easier for him to open them and look at me - and so he did! He opened his eyes very wide and looked at me, with a slight smile lighting up his face.

My mother and the Rev. PS were with us. PS, as soon as she heard that RT was sinking, had cancelled her appointments to be at my side. She anointed RT and prayed.

The doctor asked me to talk to her in the next room. She told me that she thought RT would fight on for another two days. She also told me that she had got permission for the Death Certificate to say simply 'bronchopneumonia' with no mention of HIV or AIDS. A confidential letter would go to the Coroner and that was all that was required. I thanked her and returned to RT.

I told him what she had said. I explained that I didn't want him to suffer any more. There was no need to go through the agony of another blanket bath - he could just let go. I reassured him that the doctor had promised - definitely only 'bronchopneumonia' on the Death Certificate.

As I said this, he seemed to relax and slowly his breathing changed. It became rougher and shallower. His forehead became blotchy as the circulation started to fail.

The staff nurse noticed the change. She stood close behind me with her hands on my shoulders as I held RT's hand and stroked his face.

His breathing became irregular - a long silent pause, then a few more noisy breaths - another pause - and then another -

And then it just stopped.

Epilogue

If this life is nothing more than a cruel joke; if there is no meaning behind all the suffering; if blind chance determines the manner of our lives and deaths; if it was a pointless lottery that created the scene I can never forget - of RT lying in the back of the car, screaming with agony as a small, hard turd had become wedged in his anus amongst that painful, weeping mess of undiagnosed herpes and thrush; if we are nothing more than by-products of Nature's unthinking game of genetic roulette, then I want no more of it. Life is not worth the suffering.

But I do not believe it. I know there is more. We are each of us on a journey, a voyage of discovery, learning those lessons that we most need. We cannot understand the necessity for such a hard school but there is reason behind the chaos. We do learn to overcome even the most difficult hurdles. We do find the strength, both physical and emotional, to cope with the unthinkable.

I do not understand Life any more than a small child at primary school can comprehend the arguments of a doctoral thesis. But, like that child, I can trust that there are others, older and wiser, who do know why we are here.

RT died as he wished, holding my hand. We could not be at home but we were surrounded by loving friends. Then they left us alone.

The room was quiet. RT's pain, that had filled my life for so long, had evaporated. The body seemed just an empty shell as I gently kissed him goodbye.

And yet he was still there. I could feel his presence in the room. Perhaps I had read too many tales of people who had 'died', left their bodies for a while and then 'come back to life'. It may have been imagination or wishful thinking, but I knew that RT was still with me, watching, caring.

I talked to him, told him not to worry about me, that I would be all right. I explained that it was time for him to move on - but I knew his spirit would not leave that room until I had gone home.

I went out to the Concourse to find my mother and Rev. PS. As I reached them the Lovely AR came through the front door carrying flowers. She could see from my face what had happened. As I tried to explain, the tears started to flow.

Over tea Matron explained what would happen next. The Medical Certificate of Cause of Death was being prepared. An appointment was made for me to take the certificate to the Registrar in half-an-hour. The Funeral Director was contacted and he would come to the Hospice in two hours time. There were several leaflets to read on what to do after a death.

The certificate arrived. The cause of death was given as bronchopneumonia.

I went alone to see the Registrar. She was kind and efficient. The Medical Certificate showed that RT's death had been referred to the Coroner and confirmation from that office would be required before the Death Certificate could be issued. I thought this must mean a delay of several days but a brief phone call sufficed. I assume the Hospice had sent the necessary information by fax.

Now I had two copies of that Death Certificate that had caused RT so much anxiety. As promised, there was no mention of HIV or AIDS. I returned to the Hospice to pack our things and wait for the Funeral Director.

RT's spirit still seemed to hover over me as I gathered our clothes, books and all the accumulated bits and pieces of our month of residence. His body, though warm, was no longer relevant as I said goodbye once more.

The undertaker arrived promptly, established the essential facts and arranged to telephone me that evening to confirm the date of the funeral. He would visit me at home in a few days to finalise all the arrangements.

And so, after a few emotional farewells, I was free to return home with my mother. But I didn't have a home. The builders were still in occupation. The kitchen was a bare, cold space. The other rooms were piled high with kitchen equipment and thick dust covered everything. Water and electricity had been disconnected. I would stay with my mother tonight.

My first duty was to ring my mother-in-law. She guessed what had happened as soon as she heard my voice. Then I had to think who else needed to be notified. The grapevine worked fast and the phone rang constantly.

Exhaustion drove me to sleep but I woke in the early hours. My mother heard me cough and made us some tea. Nothing seemed real.

For so long I had lived with the knowledge that RT would die. I had imagined this time over and over again. But it had always been a part of the future, not the present. But that future was now - and it made no sense. I retreated to my Mind World, that waking dream where RT waited for me, and was able to get back to sleep for a while.

The next day was filled with writing official letters, filling forms and getting my bedroom clean enough to sleep in. The builders had reconnected the water and electricity and then disappeared without explanation. I was not to see them again for two weeks.

All the stair rails, bath rails and extra steps had been fitted while we were away. As I tidied the bed I touched a button and the head of the bed rose up with a whirring sound. Now all this would have to be removed. It had arrived too late.

The Rev. R came to sort out the funeral arrangements. He had promised RT that there would be room for him to be buried in the grounds of our beautiful, Norman church on the cliff-top.

I had not yet given any thought to the nature of the service but, as we talked, I knew exactly what RT wanted - it was as though he was putting thoughts into my mind. There would be no hymns. No music at all other than the tape of that wonderful *Spem in alium* that we loved so much. It is twelve minutes long and the congregation could sit and listen while recalling their own memories of the RT that they knew.

Then I thought of the famous poem *If* by Rudyard Kipling. It encapsulates perfectly everything that RT stood for - the code by which he tried to live, and failed, as we all must fail. The vicar agreed enthusiastically with my suggestions and added some ideas of his own for prayers and readings that would, I know, have met with RT's approval.

I mentioned that the Rev. PS would be attending the funeral and the vicar immediately decided to invite her to join him in conducting the service. There would be candles, incense, flowers. The bearers would be pub landlords and old drinking companions. The coffin would be brought in to the opening bars of Rachmaninoff's *Piano Concerto No.2*, another old favourite. More music by Thomas Tallis would accompany the procession as we left for the graveside. It would be a service of which RT could be proud.

The Funeral Director found it all hard to accept. How could there be a funeral service with no organist, no hymns? But the vicar supported my decision.

It would be very important to RT that he should be correctly dressed for the occasion. I had selected some of his favourite clothes - his MCC sweater and tie, his father's thorn-proof tweed jacket, grey flannel trousers, perfectly polished brogues and his new, red socks.

I gave them to the undertaker and asked if they would bring the coffin into the house before going to the church so that I could check that RT was properly attired. The undertaker was surprised, but agreed.

So many people wanted to come to the service that I thought the church might be full. My one fear was that the secret of RT's diagnosis might be inadvertently revealed. Some would know he had died of AIDS while others would be thinking it was leukaemia. His brother would be there and I had promised that his family would not be told the truth.

I need not have worried. It seemed that RT took control of the day. While I was lying in bed, trying to find the courage to get up and face this important event, I felt a firm, peremptory tap on my shoulder as though someone was telling me to get a move on. I looked round but could see nothing that could have touched me - not even a cat.

I went to the window to find a blizzard blowing. There had been no snow all winter - but today, of all days, it was snowing and the phone calls started. Everyone that RT wanted to keep away - those he could not trust to keep his secret, those whose professional role with this disease might be recognised, those who might ask too many questions - they were all snowed in. Others, living in the same areas, were able to make the journey safely

The funeral car arrived on time and the coffin was carried into my mother's house. The undertaker asked us to wait in another room while he opened the coffin. Then I was allowed some time alone with RT.

Apart from his clothes, he looked just the same as when I left him at the Hospice more than a week ago. His face was so thin - and the cut on his forehead had not had a chance to even start to heal. But he seemed peaceful.

Suddenly all the lights started to flash and flicker. Was it the blizzard? Storms did not usually have that effect.

I adjusted his tie, tucked a copy of the poem If into his breast pocket and kissed him farewell. The undertaker replaced the lid and the lights ceased their flickering.

As we arrived at the church the snow stopped falling but it was still so bitterly cold that the bearers had to keep on their assorted, bright anoraks over their dark suits. As I followed the coffin a sudden gust of wind blew my flowers off the lid - his mother's wreath did not move at all. I stretched forward, all dignity gone, and managed to catch them before they reached the ground. Under my breath I told RT to stop fooling around, but I had to smile. It was such a typical RT joke.

The service was very moving and went exactly as planned, except for the wind that kept rattling the heavy door in the moments of silence. The voices of the two vicars, male and female, both skilled performers, complemented each other beautifully.

The music of Thomas Tallis filled the ancient building and, I am sure, there was not a dry eye in the house when those boy soprano voices soared to the rafters.

As the procession set out for the graveside the wind dropped. The undertaker had decreed that I should walk alone but Rev. PS came beside me and held my hand firmly as I fought to stay calm.

A few Words of Committal and the service was done. I threw a flower into the grave and as I turned to go home the wind returned and sleet fell. Everyone had to rush for their cars before I could give proper directions - they would follow each other to my mother's house.

But again RT seemed to take control. Some followed the wrong car and got lost, others were delayed and arrived late. At no time was the house so full that I could not keep track of the conversations and steer them away from dangerous topics such as leukaemia.

It was a good day. There were friends I had not seen since before RT became ill. Some who I had not contacted because they lived so far away had, nevertheless, heard the news and made the effort to be with me that day. There was a feeling of warmth and security in the presence of so many familiar, friendly faces.

RT's mother had not been able to come to the funeral. I had asked the undertaker to take photographs during the service and, later in the day, I returned to the grave to take some pictures of the flowers.

These I sent to my mother-in-law together with a tape of the music and copies of the prayers, psalm and poems. We talked at great length on the phone and I think she did not feel excluded from the ceremony.

There was so much to be done - letters to be answered, bureaucracy to be satisfied, clothes to be sorted, papers to be read and filed or destroyed. I was aware that I was treading a tightrope, that I must fight to keep my balance.

On one side was the Slough of Despond, the trap of wallowing in emotion, allowing myself to sink into despair and loneliness. On the other was the temptation to throw myself into furious activity, to stop myself from thinking, to run away from the pain.

Somehow I had to find the balance that was right for me, that would let me progress into my new future without losing all that was valuable in my life with RT.

I found myself searching for photographs. As a journalist RT had taken thousands and in those dusty boxes, amongst pictures of boats, fishermen and seascapes, were occasional shots of him - as a child and a youth as well as the more recent pictures.

Every day I searched a different box, desperate to find these little pieces of his life. I felt that if only I could gather enough bits of him together I would discover the magic word that would, inevitably, bring him back to life.

The past seemed so close that I was sure there must be a way to turn the clock back. I could not believe that he was really gone. He looked so alive in all those photographs. He could not have ceased to exist.

I stuck photos up all over the house so that I could talk to him all the time. Whenever I went to bed I could meet him in the Mind World for a cuddle before falling into the sleep of emotional exhaustion. Every book of his that I picked up seemed to fall open at an appropriate passage about constant wives or holding on to memories.

One, a little French fairy story book that I had never seen before, opened at a picture of a woman standing by an open window. The caption read, 'And she heard a voice on the wind, crying, "Have you forgotten your husband who loves you and is waiting for you?" ' I felt that RT was there, beside me, trying to communicate - but it was not enough. I wanted him, alive, not just his spirit.

The Community Care Nurse came round once to make sure that I was coping. He was planning to establish a support group in the city and hoped that I would become involved.

He asked, as all the professionals asked, what did I want or need? I could not answer him but, as soon as he had gone, I was able to write my answer:-

What do I want?

> *I want someone to stop the pain, to tell me that everything is all right, that he will soon be home again, that this is all a dream.*
> *I want to be held and comforted - preferably by him.*
> *I want to talk about the past two years.*
> *I want to feel better.*

What do I need?

> *I don't know - I've never been here before.*
> *I don't know what helps or who.*
> *I know I need help but what does that mean?*

Talking helped. Now I no longer had to maintain such secrecy. I would try to keep RT's family from learning the truth if I could but, as I intended to start campaigning for AIDS awareness and to help those organisations that had been so supportive to us over the past months, word would soon spread amongst my friends.

To those that I knew I could trust I now turned. I needed to tell people about the pain of the past two years. I had to express some of those thoughts, memories and feelings that were filling my mind and preventing me from learning how to live without RT.

Crying didn't help, though I never tried to stop the tears when I was alone. But when the crying was done the pain was still there.

Helping others with their pain and trouble helped me. When I could listen to others who were suffering the same torments I had experienced and offer my support and understanding then I found a purpose to my life again.

Going back to the Hospice did help. I needed to make sure that RT was not still there waiting for me. I needed to see all those familiar faces again to know for certain that it had not been some long, strange dream.

Reading books about Near Death Experiences and other peoples beliefs helped me to clarify my own ideas and faith. Reading obituaries filled me with envy. Those lucky people had already moved on, gone home - when would it be my turn? Would RT be there to greet me? How long must I stay here?

Writing helped most of all. I knew that RT had wanted me to write his book but I did not know where to start. I thought I would wait a few months until I felt stronger. But just four weeks after RT died an image of the first page appeared in my mind. I could see it clearly and read the words. Something was forcing me to write it down. And then I could not stop. I had to keep on writing.

With the writing came the memories. I could see RT lying in bed with his agonisingly sore bottom exposed to the air. I could see him, naked and drunk, sprawled upside down on our narrow, winding staircase, unable to move. I could see him in his wheelchair, laughing as I sped with him, dangerously, down the centre of the road.

I could feel the exhaustion of being woken for perhaps the third time that night by RT demanding yet another set of bedclothes as a drenching sweat had soaked the bed again. Or the frustration of making tea at 3am only to find that RT had already gone back to sleep. The despair of watching rainwater stream in under the kitchen door.

I remembered the hours spent sitting quietly together in pubs, sometimes managing a gentle game of pool or billiards. And that awful day, holding hands in shocked silence until RT made his dutiful proposal.

I remember with joy his surprised delight when he realised that we were married and that he loved me; the pride with which he introduced me everywhere as his 'wife'; the difficulty I had in persuading him not to wear a full, formal morning suit and grey topper for the intimate, brief Registry Office wedding.

There were the cosy evenings spent watching videos of John Betjeman over and over again. The fun of introducing RT to all the Marx Brothers' films. The hours of talking. The gentle intimacy of lying beside him and massaging his back and limbs until he fell asleep. The wonderful time when he found the strength to massage my head to help ease my distress.

There were nights of unreasoning rage when only our cats dare approach him, forcing him to calm down as they demanded to be stroked.

Hours of fear and loneliness at night and during the long weekends when only an emergency could justify a call to a doctor or a nurse.

The Convent holds many happy memories - of strawberries, hugs and kisses; talking to fellow sufferers; eating well; RT's love of his female therapists; walking or sitting in the gardens.

And our own gardens - created with so much love and effort. The slate walls and raised beds full of shrubs. The little crooked greenhouse we constructed out of scrap, that survived so many storms unscathed but that now, no longer needed, collapsed in the gales at the time of the funeral.

So many memories from such few short years - from when we first started working together writing and publishing our own magazine and newspaper to that last morning when RT looked at me and whispered, "Hallo."

Was there a point to it all? Is there a reason for the pain? Did we learn anything?

There was one day when RT turned to me and said, his voice full of wonder and surprise, "You are the first person in my life to really love me for myself and not for what I can give!"

Since childhood he had trained himself to be the charming companion, to make sure that he kept his friends entertained. It was a role that worked for him.

He had many friends but felt that he could never risk allowing his mask to slip. In earlier relationships he had discovered that failure to hide his true feelings would lead to rejection. Now, at last, he felt safe enough to express his anger, fear and pain, to lose his dignity and let that stiff upper lip tremble.

He knew that my love was strong enough to survive all the drunken rows and terrified tantrums. He trusted me to understand and forgive, to help him through his mental torment and to stand by him - to be 'on his side' at all times.

It was not easy. I hated the person he became when alcohol took control. I was frightened of his unreasoning rage. I could not cope with the illogicality of his arguments and despised his long periods of total selfishness and self-pity.

But I learnt that I could survive, could forgive. I learnt to fight back, to shout and argue, to walk away when he was at his most impossible. I learnt to love.

And now, as I try to start to live the rest of my life, the time has come . . . I must be tested. I need to know. Am I HIV+?

Do I have 'it'?

Postscript

Three months after RT died my work, unexpectedly, took me to the tiny village next to that holy well and chapel we had visited last summer. I bought some red ribbon and drove to the car park.

It had been raining all day but, as I got out of the car, the rain stopped and the sun managed to break through the clouds. The car park was deserted and I felt utterly alone as I set off to walk down the narrow woodland path towards the well. What was I doing here? Why had I come?

To break the overwhelming silence I spoke, softly, "RT - are you there?" and, just beside me, a large leaf slowly waved up and down. Nothing else moved.

I walked on a little further, refusing to believe this foolish coincidence. Then I simply had to ask again, "Are you there?" and once again a single leaf moved up and down.

This was ridiculous. It was probably just a mouse or a bird brushing against the plants. And yet, I had to ask just once more, "Are you really with me?" and again a single leaf moved decisively, quite vigorously, up and down. This time I accepted the sign. I believed that, somehow, RT was here, at my side, willing me to make this brief pilgrimage to a holy place that he had loved.

I climbed over the ancient stone stile and approached the muddy pool that was the holy well. The overhanging branches were still covered with the ribbons I had remembered so vividly. I stretched across to reach a thick branch near the centre of the pool where I tied a red ribbon for RT. Then I continued along the path towards the chapel ruins.

A large fir tree was spreading its sheltering branches above the ancient stone altar. I climbed up to it and tied another ribbon for RT. In one corner of the chapel a stream bubbled into the natural font. Here I knelt to touch the water and tossed in a small coin to join the many others lying below. It seemed the right thing to do. A tiny gesture to the spirits that so clearly guarded this holy place.

I left the chapel, retracing my steps to the sacred pool and, again, added a coin to all the other offerings that had been left there. My task was finished. All I could do now was to make my lonely way back to the car. I felt miserable. Why had I come? Was it just to fulfil the prophecy that I had made on that earlier visit - that I would come here again but that I would be alone?

Slowly, sadly, I turned to the old stone stile. And there, on the step where I had placed my foot just a few minutes ago, was a tiny violet, freshly plucked, root and all, absolutely perfect. How had it come there? It was so delicate - it can only have lain there for a few moments. It certainly had not been there before - I would have trodden on it as I climbed down towards the pool.

Carefully, I picked the flower up and cradled it in my hands, wondering. Still, there was no one else around. I returned to the car park and that, too, was still deserted. I knew that there had been no other visitors to the well while I was there.

Sitting in the car, I opened my diary and gently placed the beautiful little violet inside. I would treasure this final gift from RT.

As I drove away, returning to reality, I understood why I had been called back to this special place. I looked towards that woodland path and whispered, . . .

. . . "Thank you, my love."

Appendix

USEFUL PUBLICATIONS

Nick Bamforth
AIDS and the Healer Within, Amethyst Books, 1987

Leon Chaitow
Candida Albicans, Thorsons, 1985

Vicky Cosstick, editor
AIDS - Meeting the Community Challenge, St Paul Publications, 1987

Thorwald Dethlefsen & Rüdiger Dahlke, M.D.
The Healing Power of Illness, Element Books, 1983

Betty Eadie
Embraced By The Light, Thorsons, 1994

Ursula Fleming
Grasping the Nettle, Collins, 1990

Louise L. Hay
You Can Heal Your Life, Eden Grove Editions, 1984
The AIDS Book, Hay House, 1988

John W. James & Frank Cherry
The Grief Recovery Handbook, Harper Perennial, 1988

Debra Jarvis
HIV Positive, Lion Publishing, 1990

Elisabeth Kübler-Ross, M.D.
On Death and Dying, Collier Books, 1970
Death - The Final Stage of Growth, Simon & Schuster, 1975
AIDS - The Ultimate Challenge, Macmillan, 1987
On Life After Death, Celestial Arts, 1991

Mary Mortimer
When Your Partner Dies, The Women's Press, 1995

National AIDS Manual
HIV & AIDS Treatment Directory, NAM Publications, annual
AIDS Treatment Update, NAM Publications monthly

Neil McNicholas
Death - A Friendly Companion, CTS Publications, 1992

Palinurus (Cyril Connolly)
The Unquiet Grave, Hamish Hamilton, 1945

Jenifer Pardoe
How Many Times Can You Say Goodbye?, Triangle, SPCK, 1991

M. Scott Peck
The Road Less Travelled, Simon & Schuster, 1978

Laura Pinsky & Paul Harding Douglas with Craig Metroka, M.D., Ph.D.
The Essential HIV Treatment Fact Book, Pocket Books, 1992

Mel Pohl, M.D., Deniston Kay, Ph.D. & Doug Toft
The Caregivers' Journey, Hazelden Foundation, 1990

Ines Rieder & Patricia Ruppelt
Matters of Life and Death - Women speak about AIDS, Virago, 1988

D. Scott Rogo
The Return from Silence, The Aquarian Press, 1989

Dr. G. Edward Rozar, Jr.
Laughing in the Face of AIDS, Baker Book House, 1992

Betty Shine
Mind Magic, Corgi Books, 1991

Trevor Smith, M.A.,M.B.,BChir,D.P.M.,M.F.Hom.
Homoeopathic Medicine, Thorsons, 1982

Harald Tietze
Kombucha - The Miracle Fungus, Gateway Books, 1995

Robert G. Twycross,M.A.,D.M.,F.R.C.P. & Sylvia A. Lack,M.B.,B.S.
Oral Morphine, Beaconsfield, 1987

Frances Vaughan & Roger Walsh - editors
A Gift of Healing - (Selections from A Course in Miracles), Arkana, 1990

Colin Wilson
Afterlife, Grafton Books, 1987

USEFUL ADDRESSES

BODY POSITIVE
51b Philbeach Gardens, London SW5 9EB   0171 373 9124
Self-help group for people living with or directly affected by HIV/AIDS

EQUILIBRIUM
BM Equilibrium, London WC1N 3XX   0171 226 8536
Treatment Journal produced by and for people affected by HIV and AIDS

NATIONAL AIDS HELPLINE
PO Box 5000, Glasgow G12 9JQ   0800 561123
A 24 hour national helpline for confidential advice and information

NAM PUBLICATIONS
16a Clapham Common, Southside, London SW4 7AB 0171 627 3200
Comprehensive and up-to-date publications on HIV/AIDS treatments

THE TERENCE HIGGINS TRUST (THT)
52-54 Grays Inn Road, London WC1X 8JU   0171 831 0330
Helpline for advice and information - daily 12noon - 10pm   *0171 242 1010*